Pocket Anatomy
& Protocols for
Abdominal
Ultrasound

T0200969

To My Author and Creator:
Thank you for your abounding love, unmerited favor,
and the ability to share knowledge.

To Lisa, Devin, and Reagan:
Thank you for the love, joy, and support you provide
me with daily. I love you.

Sandra Broadhead, RDMS, RT(R)
Sonographer, Alta View Hospital
Sandy, Utah
Graduate, Weber State University
Ogden, Utah

Krista Downey, ARDMS, ARRT
Graduate
Weber State University
Ogden, Utah
Graduate
Utah State University
Logan, Utah

Traci B. Fox, EdD, RT(R), RDMS, RVT
Associate Professor
Department of Medical Imaging and Radiation Sciences
Thomas Jefferson University
Philadelphia, Pennsylvania

Martie Grant, MEd
Faculty, Diagnostic Medical Sonography Program
Northern Alberta Institute of Technology
Edmonton, Alberta, Canada

Jennifer Myers, RDMS, RT(R)
Student
Department of Medical Imaging and Radiologic Sciences
College of Health Professionals
Thomas Jefferson University
Philadelphia, Pennsylvania

Danika Ashley Washington, BS, AAS
Diagnostic Medical Sonographer
United States Airforce
Keesler Air Force Base, Mississippi

Diagnostic medical sonography has become an imaging modality that is utilized regularly, not only as a screening tool, but as an investigative instrument that can identify abnormalities of the abdomen and small parts, and thus positively influencing the clinical course of many of our patients. At the core of our clinical practice lies the establishment of a thorough imaging protocol, a protocol that not only demonstrates normal sonographic anatomy, but also affords the practitioner the ability to recognize anatomic variants and, most importantly, pathologic conditions. This book has been created for, and will mostly serve those with minimal sonography experience, best. Thus, sonography students and other medical students will appreciate its format and structure. But it can also serve the advanced practitioner as a reference guide and a quick review of normal sonographic anatomy and physiology as well. Accordingly, the primary goal of *Pocket Anatomy & Protocols for Abdominal Ultrasound* is to offer the sonographic imager a readily accessible resource that assists with clinical assessment, protocol establishment, and the identification of normal sonographic anatomy.

HOW TO USE THIS POCKET BOOK

Each chapter in this small in size, though information-packed, resource is created with clinical practice in mind. Consequently, this book can be used prior to beginning an exam as a review of imaging requirements, clinical questions, sonographic anatomy, and protocol suggestions. During the exam, one can return to its pages for insight and assistance. After the exam, it can be utilized as a reference for normal measurements, common pathology, and image correlation. The following suggested steps are also provided to offer a means whereby one can maximize the utilization of this resource appropriately in the clinical setting.

STEP #1: POCKET IT!

We have created this book to fit in the clinical setting. Therefore, put this book in a pocket or have it readily available on a shelf nearby so that you can use it as a resource if needed. If space allows, it could even be placed on the ultrasound system for quick access.

STEP #2: REVIEW NORMAL ANATOMY AND PHYSIOLOGY

Though the purpose of this book is not to offer a thorough anatomy and physiology review of each organ or structure, it does contain enough information to provide a quick recap of anatomy and physiology for each organ or structure prior to sonographic analysis. Anatomic drawings are provided as well.

STEP #3: REVIEW PATIENT PREPARATION AND SUGGESTED EQUIPMENT

This book provides some patient preparation information and positioning techniques that may be useful. Also, it offers equipment suggestions, including transducer types and frequencies to employ for optimal image quality. Prior to the exam beginning, be sure to have all equipment in optimal working condition in order to ensure safe and accurate patient care.

STEP #4: REVIEW NORMAL SONOGRAPHIC ANATOMY

Briefly review normal sonographic anatomy. Though you will expectantly have the book with you, a preemptive quick anatomic review over normal sonographic appearances and anatomy would be beneficial. Short video clips of sonographic anatomy are provided online for you as well.

STEP #5: REVIEW THE SUGGESTED PROTOCOL

The American Institute of Ultrasound in Medicine (AIUM), in conjunction with other medical organizations, works to establish indications and recommendations for sonographic imaging. In each chapter, AIUM-specific recommendations for individual abdominal structures are offered. With these recommendations in mind, a fundamental protocol has been provided in each chapter. Nonetheless, we recognize that protocols vary between medical institutions, and thus alterations may be required to our suggested construct. However, the protocols contained herein will prospectively provide a fundamental groundwork, upon which additions or subtractions can be made by the practitioner in conjunction with previously established routines and advancements in future technology.

STEP #6: CLINICAL INVESTIGATION

An important role of the sonographer is the obligation to obtain a thorough clinical history. In each chapter, specific clinical history questions are provided. If these questions are asked prior to commencing the examination, they will hopefully help one establish a clinically focused evaluation, resulting in individualized examination-specific protocol adjustments and a more tailored sonographic study.

STEP #7: PERFORMING THE EXAMINATION

Refer to the pages of this book throughout the examination when needed for sonographic anatomy, scanning tips, a "where else to look" section for each topic, and normal measurements.

STEP #8: ESSENTIAL PATHOLOGY FOCUS

Lastly, although this is not a sonographic pathology textbook, some most common pathologies, including clinical history related to those pathologies and images, are provided in this book. The list of pathologies is not extensive in order to encourage the portability of the text, so we suggest having additional pathology-focused materials nearby in this regard.

FINAL WORDS

With ever-evolving changes and advancements in medicine, it is our obligation as medical professionals to stay abreast of specialized recommendations, imaging requirements, and protocol additions that can often dramatically improve patient care. And although this book provides a much-needed fundamental clinical reference, it is incumbent upon us all to continue to learn more and work to exploit, to the best of our ability, the irreplaceable uses of ultrasound in medicine as we care for our patients. Thank you for choosing this book as a resource. I pray that *Pocket Anatomy & Protocols for Abdominal Ultrasound* serves you and your patients well.

Steven M. Penny

I would first like to thank my family for allowing me the time away from them to work on this project. Thanks must also be offered to my editorial team and the staff at Wolters Kluwer, especially Sharon Zinner, Eric McDermott, and Caroline Define, for their encouragement and guidance throughout this new project. I am also grateful to my coworkers at Johnston Community College and my past and current students for the daily interaction that require me to continually learn, providing me with intellectual stimulation and the need for professional growth. Lastly, I would like to express gratitude to those who have chosen to work in the noble profession of diagnostic medical sonography—my colleagues—for constantly pursuing excellence and for providing instrumental vital patient care all over the world.

CONTENTS

CHAPTER 1

Abdominal Sonography Overview

INTRODUCTION

This brief overview chapter provides information pertaining to the AIUM indications for a sonogram of the abdomen and/or the retroperitoneum. General sonographic terminology, patient positioning, and common sonographic artifacts are provided. Furthermore, a summary chart of abnormal laboratory findings and possible sonographic pathologies is presented. This chapter also includes a summary of the focused assessment with sonography for trauma (FAST) examination and a reminder to practice proper body mechanics while performing sonographic examinations in order to reduce the likelihood of work-related musculoskeletal disorders.

AIUM INDICATIONS FOR AN ABDOMEN AND/OR RETROPERITONEUM SONOGRAM[1]

- Abdominal, flank, and/or back pain.
- Signs or symptoms that may be referred from the abdominal and/or retroperitoneal regions, such as jaundice or hematuria.
- Palpable abnormalities such as an abdominal mass or organomegaly.
- Abnormal laboratory values or abnormal findings on other imaging examinations suggestive of abdominal and/or retroperitoneal pathology.
- Follow-up of known or suspected abnormalities in the abdomen and/or retroperitoneum.
- Search for metastatic disease or an occult primary neoplasm.
- Evaluation of cirrhosis, portal hypertension, and transjugular intrahepatic portosystemic shunt (TIPS) stents; screening for

hepatoma; and evaluation of the liver in conjunction with liver elastography.
- Abdominal trauma.
- Evaluation of urinary tract infection and hydronephrosis.
- Evaluation of uncontrolled hypertension and suspected renal artery stenosis.
- Search for the presence of free or loculated peritoneal and/or retroperitoneal fluid.
- Evaluation of suspected congenital abnormalities.
- Evaluation of suspected hypertrophic pyloric stenosis, intussusception, necrotizing enterocolitis, or any other bowel abnormalities.
- Pretransplantation and posttransplantation evaluation.
- Planning for and guiding an invasive procedure.

EQUIPMENT SELECTION AND QUALITY CONTROL[1]

- Ultrasound equipment will naturally vary between institutions.
- It is the institution's obligation to offer high-quality sonographic examinations, and therefore these providers should consequently supply equipment that balances sensibility and state-of-the-art features for their sonographic practitioners to utilize.
- Institutions should be mindful of the potential for practitioner musculoskeletal injuries and thus should purchase equipment that encourages the use of correct ergonomics.
- Ultrasound machines should be capable of standard real-time imaging, have color, power, and spectral Doppler abilities, and be capable of providing diagnostic images for interpretation by a certified interpreting physician.
- Curved sector transducers and/or linear transducers are commonly utilized for abdominal and retroperitoneal sonography (Fig. 1-1).
- For most preadolescent pediatric patients, mean frequencies of 5 MHz or greater are preferred, and in neonates and small infants, a higher-frequency transducer is often necessary.
- For adults, mean frequencies between 4 and 6 MHz are most commonly used.

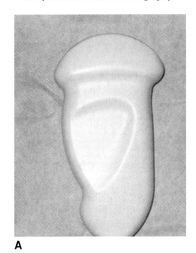

A

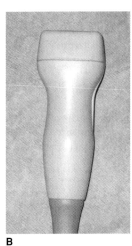

B

Figure 1-1. Transducers for abdominal imaging. A: Curvilinear array. Curvilinear, curved, or convex array transducer. Used commonly in abdominal examinations. B: Linear phased array transducer may be used for superficial abdominal imaging and some gastrointestinal studies as well. (Part A adapted with permission from Penny S, Fox T, Godwin CH, eds. *Examination Review for Ultrasound: Sonographic Principles & Instrumentation.* Philadelphia, PA: Wolters Kluwer Health/Lippincott Williams & Wilkins; 2011. Part B reprinted with permission from Penny SM, ed. *Introduction to Sonography and Patient Care.* Philadelphia, PA: Wolters Kluwer; 2015.)

- Higher frequencies, including the use of a linear transducer, are often used and needed when evaluating the abdominal wall, liver surface, and bowel.
- Quality control and improvement, safety, infection control, patient education, and equipment performance monitoring should be in accordance with the AIUM *Standards and Guidelines for the Accreditation of Ultrasound Practices* found at https://www.aium.org/accreditation/accreditation.aspx

THE ALARA PRINCIPLE[1]

- Sonography should be practiced by trained health care practitioners.
- According to the AIUM, "The potential benefits and risks of each examination should be considered. The ALARA (as low as reasonably achievable) principle should be observed when adjusting controls that affect the acoustic output and by considering transducer dwell times."
- Sonographers should strive for image optimization, while simultaneously minimizing total ultrasound exposure in order to practice the ALARA principle.

SONOGRAPHIC TERMINOLOGY[2]

- Common sonographic descriptive terms are provided in **Table 1-1.**
- Keep in mind, the normal echogenicity of the abdominal organs from brightest to darkest are as follows: renal sinus, pancreas, spleen, liver, renal cortex, renal pyramid, and gallbladder.

| Table 1-1 | SONOGRAPHIC TERMS AND A BRIEF EXPLANATION |

SONOGRAPHIC DESCRIPTIVE TERM	EXPLANATION
Anechoic	Without echoes
Complex	Consists of both solid and cystic components
Echogenic	Structure that produces echoes; often used as a comparative term
Heterogeneous	Of differing composition
Homogeneous	Of uniform composition
Hyperechoic	Having many echoes
Hypoechoic	Having few echoes
Isoechoic	Having the same echogenicity

1. Abdominal Sonography

COMMON ARTIFACTS[2,3]

- Ultrasound artifacts abound during sonographic imaging, with several of them providing useful diagnostic information (Table 1-2).

Table 1-2   COMMON ULTRASOUND ARTIFACTS

ARTIFACT	DESCRIPTION
Acoustic shadowing (Fig. 1-2)	Occurs when sound encounters a high attenuator
Comet tail (Fig. 1-3)	Type of reverberation artifact caused by small structures
Dirty shadowing (Fig. 1-4)	Acoustic shadowing containing reverberation artifact
Edge shadowing (Fig. 1-5)	Sound refracts off of round surfaces
Mirror image	Occurs when sound reflects off of a strong reflector and creates a duplicate of the anatomy which can be seen deeper in the image
Posterior enhancement (through transmission) (Fig. 1-6)	Occurs when sound encounters a weak attenuator
Refraction (Fig. 1-7)	Causes the duplication of anatomy because of the sound beam striking an interface at nonperpendicular angles
Reverberation (Fig. 1-8)	Bouncing of the sound beam between two or more interfaces
Ring-down (Fig. 1-9)	Caused by sound interacting with small air bubbles causing the bubbles to vibrate

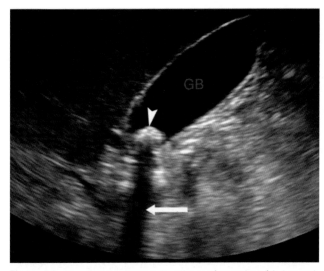

Figure 1-2. Acoustic shadowing. A gallstone (*arrowhead*) is located in the neck of the gallbladder (*GB*) producing an acoustic shadow (*arrow*). (Reprinted with permission from Klein J, Pohl J, Vinson EN, Brant WE, Helms CA, eds. *Brant and Helms' Fundamentals of Diagnostic Radiology.* 5th ed. Philadelphia, PA: Wolters Kluwer; 2018.)

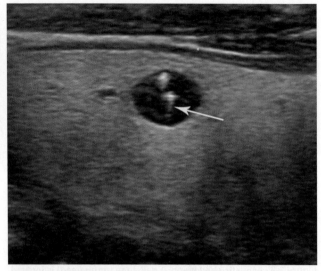

Figure 1-3. Comet tail artifact. A sharply defined cystic lesion within the right thyroid lobe shows floating punctate echogenic foci with a tapering tail (*arrow*). (Reprinted with permission from Brant WE, Helms C, eds. *Fundamentals of Diagnostic Radiology*. 4th ed. Philadelphia, PA: Wolters Kluwer Health/Lippincott Williams & Wilkins; 2012.)

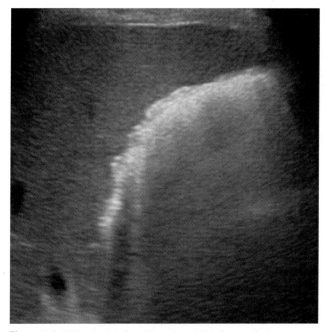

Figure 1-4. Dirty shadowing. Dirty shadowing is noted emanating from the emphysematous gallbladder wall that contains air.
(Reprinted with permission from Hsu WC, Cummings FP, eds. *Gastrointestinal Imaging: A Core Review*. Philadelphia, PA: Wolters Kluwer; 2016.)

1. Abdominal Sonography

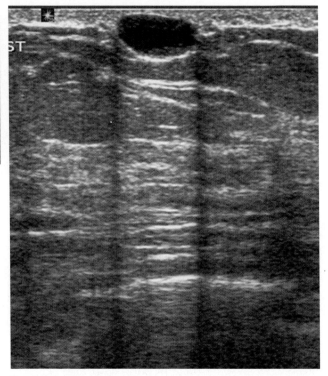

Figure 1-5. Edge shadowing. Distinct shadowing can be seen emanating from the edge of this cyst. (Reprinted with permission from Shirkhoda A, ed. *Variants and Pitfalls in Body Imaging.* 2nd ed. Philadelphia, PA: Wolters Kluwer Health/Lippincott Williams & Wilkins; 2010.)

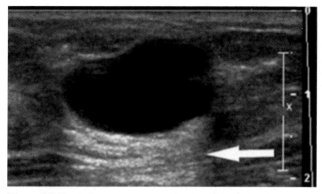

Figure 1-6. Posterior enhancement. Posterior enhancement, also referred as through transmission, is seen (*arrow*) posterior to this cyst. (Reprinted with permission from Klein J, Pohl J, Vinson EN, Brant WE, Helms CA, eds. *Brant and Helms' Fundamentals of Diagnostic Radiology.* 5th ed. Philadelphia, PA: Wolters Kluwer; 2018.)

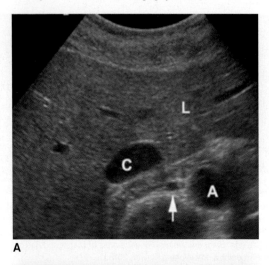

A

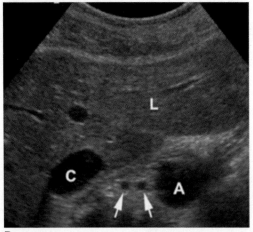

B

Figure 1-7. **Refraction artifact. A: Transverse view of the upper abdomen with the transducer positioned lateral to the midline shows the left lobe of the liver (*L*), aorta (*A*), vena cava (*C*), and a single azygos vein (*arrow*). B: With the transducer positioned in the midline, rectus muscle refraction has resulted in duplication of the azygos vein (*arrows*).** (Reprinted with permission from Siegel MJ, ed. *Pediatric Sonography*. 4th ed. Philadelphia, PA: Wolters Kluwer Health/ Lippincott Williams & Wilkins; 2010.)

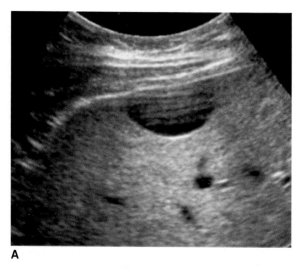

A

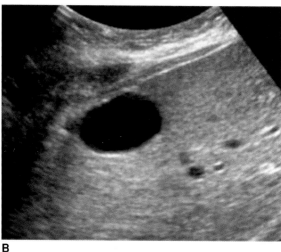

B

Figure 1-8. Reverberation. A: View of a hepatic cyst shows multiple reverberation echoes filling much of the lumen of the cyst. B: By repositioning the transducer so that the cyst is deeper in the image, the reverberation artifacts are eliminated and the cyst is entirely anechoic. (Reprinted with permission from Siegel MJ, ed. *Pediatric Sonography.* 4th ed. Philadelphia, PA: Wolters Kluwer Health/Lippincott Williams & Wilkins; 2010.)

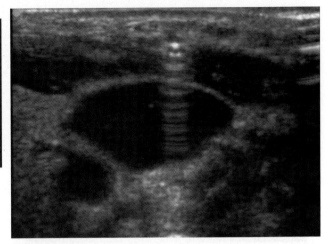

Figure 1-9. Ring-down artifact. Ring-down artifact noted emanating from an echogenic needle. (Reprinted with permission from Shah KH, Mason C, eds. *Essential Emergency Procedures*. 2nd ed. Philadelphia, PA: Wolters Kluwer; 2015.)

BASICS OF DOPPLER SONOGRAPHY[3]

- Color Doppler (CD) and Power Doppler (PD)
  - CD allocates varying colors to traveling red blood cells depending upon their velocity and the direction of their flow relative to the location of the transducer.
  - For most ultrasound machines, flow toward the transducer is allocated red, while flow away from the transducer is allocated blue (**Fig. 1-10**).
  - Faster speeds are typically depicted with brighter colors and slower velocities are depicted with darker colors.
  - Optimal CD imaging is obtained with oblique imaging, whereas a perpendicular orientation will be void of color.
  - In abdominal imaging, CD is often utilized to depict flow direction within vascular structures, such as the portal vein, and to identify flow within specific abdominal organs and identified masses. Increased CD within an organ or structure is indicative of hyperemia and may be a sign of inflammation or infection.
  - PD is a more sensitive form of CD (**Fig. 1-11**).

1. Abdominal Sonography

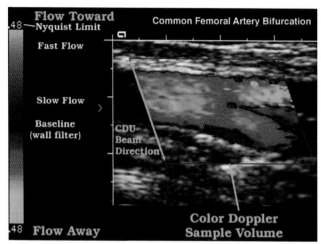

Figure 1-10. Color Doppler. The color map on the left side of the image shows *red* as the dominant color above the baseline indicating flow relatively toward the color Doppler beam direction. *Blue* is the dominant color below the color map baseline indicating flow relatively away from the color Doppler beam direction. (Reprinted with permission from Brant WE, Helms C, eds. *Fundamentals of Diagnostic Radiology.* 4th ed. Philadelphia, PA: Wolters Kluwer Health/ Lippincott Williams & Wilkins; 2012.)

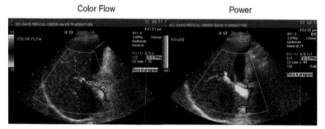

Figure 1-11. Comparison of color Doppler and power Doppler. Color Doppler (*left*) and power Doppler (*right*) studies show the enhanced sensitivity of the power Doppler acquisition, particularly in areas perpendicular to the beam direction, where the signal is lost in the color Doppler image. Flow directionality, however, is not available in the power Doppler image. (Reprinted with permission from Bushberg JT, Seibert JA, Leidholdt EM, Boone JM, eds. *Essential Physics of Medical Imaging.* 3rd ed. Philadelphia, PA: Wolters Kluwer Health/Lippincott Williams & Wilkins; 2011.)

- PD exploits the amplitude of the Doppler signal.
- PD does not typically provide flow direction.
- PD is useful in providing evidence of flow in smaller or low-flow vessels.
- Excessive motion can inhibit the effective use of PD.
- Pulsed-wave Doppler (PW)
  - PW is utilized to analyze the flow characteristics of a specific vascular structure, with the ability to evaluate a specific area within that vessel.
  - The pulsed sound is placed in a sample gate, thus providing Doppler information from the specific selected point within the chosen vessel.
  - PW can provide flow direction.
    - Flow toward the transducer is often displayed above the baseline, while flow away from the transducer is often displayed below the baseline.
    - Be sure to evaluate whether the flow direction control has been *inverted* before making a final diagnostic conclusion.
  - Flow pattern can also be analyzed with PW. Veins typically have a continuous rhythmic flow pattern in diastole and systole.
    - Arteries typically have an alternating pitch, with high peaks in systole and lower crest in systole.
  - Resistive patterns can be depicted with PW.
    - Vessels can be described as having a low- or high-resistant pattern.
      - Low-resistive patterns are depicted by a biphasic systolic peak and a comparatively high level of diastolic flow **(Fig. 1-12)**.
      - High-resistive patterns are depicted by a high systolic peak and low level of diastolic flow **(Fig. 1-13)**.
    - The resistive patterns for specific abdominal vessels can be found in the organ or structure chapters provided in this text.
- Continuous-wave Doppler (CW Doppler)
  - CW Doppler is a technique in which the sound beam is continuously emitted from one crystal, while a second crystal received the returning signal.
  - CW Doppler is not typically utilized in abdominal imaging.

1. Abdominal Sonography

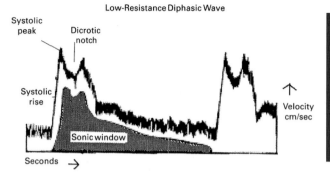

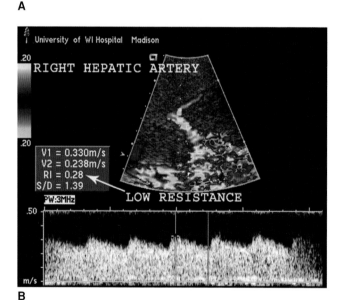

Figure 1-12. Low-resistance pattern. A: Diagram of an arterial spectral waveform in a low-resistance bed. Note the relatively high diastolic flow. B: Pulsed Doppler sonogram from a low-resistance system. (Reprinted with permission from Sanders RC, ed. *Clinical Sonography: A Practical Guide*. 5th ed. Philadelphia, PA: Wolters Kluwer; 2015.)

High-Resistance Wave

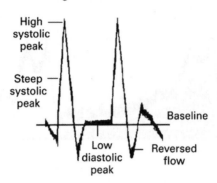

A

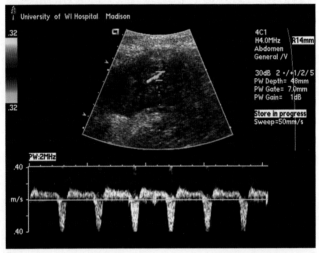

B

Figure 1-13. **High-resistance pattern. A: Diagram of an arterial spectral waveform in a high-resistance bed. B: Pulsed Doppler sonogram from a high-resistance system.** (Reprinted with permission from Sanders RC, ed. *Clinical Sonography: A Practical Guide.* 5th ed. Philadelphia, PA: Wolters Kluwer; 2015.)

GENERAL CLINICAL HISTORY QUERIES

- Why did your doctor order this sonogram? *Though some patients may be poor historians, others may be capable of providing much beneficial information regarding their current and past clinical record.*
- Where is your pain? *If possible, have the patient point with one finger to the most painful region. Assessing the area of complaint prior to an abdominal sonogram can provide some beneficial insight. **Figure 1-14** provides a helpful map with associated common pain locations for various organ and structures.*
- How long have you had pain? *This question can reveal a chronic or an acute situation.*
- Have you had any nausea or vomiting? *Nausea and vomiting can be associated with many gastrointestinal issues. If possible, inquire as to how often vomiting has occurred.*
- Are you a diabetic or have high blood pressure? *Diabetics and those suffering from high blood pressure can have related clinical issues. This is a good question to assess the overall health of the patient.*
- Have you had any recent weight loss? *Unexplained weight loss is a worrisome clinical history complaint that has been associated with some forms of cancer. Inquire as to how much weight loss has occurred and over how much time as well.*

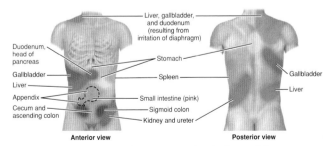

Figure 1-14. Area of pain for various abdominal complaints.
(Reprinted with permission from Moore KL, Dalley AF, Agur AM, eds. *Clinically Oriented Anatomy.* 7th ed. Philadelphia, PA: Wolters Kluwer Health/Lippincott Williams & Wilkins; 2013.)

● Have you had any relevant surgeries (specific to the organ or structures being examined)? *This question is helpful in providing a surgical history in order to establish the possible absence of organs or the existence of known deviations from normal anatomy that may be encountered during the sonographic examination.*

SUMMARY OF RELEVANT LABORATORY VALUES AND KEY ABDOMINAL FINDINGS (TABLE 1-3)[4]

Table 1-3	POSSIBLE LABORATORY FINDINGS AND POTENTIAL ABDOMINAL PATHOLOGIES
LABORATORY FINDING	**KEY ABDOMINAL FINDINGS**
↑ Alanine aminotransferase (ALT)	Biliary tract, pancreatic, or hepatic disease
↑ Alkaline phosphatase (ALP)	Biliary obstruction, liver cancer, pancreatic disease, gallstones
↑ Amylase	Pancreatitis (acute or chronic), pancreatic carcinoma, pancreatic duct or biliary duct obstruction, or gallbladder disease
↑ Aspartate aminotransferase (AST)	Pancreatic disease or liver damage
↑ Bilirubin	Liver disease, biliary obstruction, or other biliary disease
↑ Blood urea nitrogen (BUN)	Renal disease, renal obstruction, dehydration, gastrointestinal bleeding, or congestive heart failure
↑ Calcitonin	Thyroid cancer, lung cancer, and anemia
↑ Creatinine (Cr or Creat)	Renal damage, renal infection, or renal obstruction
↑ Gamma-glutamyltransferase (GGT)	Liver disease or biliary obstruction
↑ Lipase	Acute pancreatitis, gallbladder disease, or pancreatic or biliary duct obstruction

Table 1-3	**POSSIBLE LABORATORY FINDINGS AND POTENTIAL ABDOMINAL PATHOLOGIES** (*Continued*)

LABORATORY FINDING	KEY ABDOMINAL FINDINGS
↑ Partial thromboplastin time (PTT)	Liver disease, anticoagulation therapy, and hereditary coagulopathies
↑ Serum calcium	Parathyroid abnormalities
↑ Thyroid-stimulating hormone (TSH), thyroxine (T$_4$), or triiodothyronine (T$_3$)	Hyperthyroidism
↑ White blood cell (WBC)	Inflammatory disease or infection
↓ Albumin	Liver disease
↓ Alkaline phosphatase (ALP)	Wilson disease
↓ Hematocrit	Hemorrhage
↓ Partial thromboplastin time (PTT)	Vitamin K deficiency
↓ Thyroid-stimulating hormone (TSH), thyroxine (T$_4$), or triiodothyronine (T$_3$)	Hypothyroidism

1. Abdominal Sonography

PATIENT POSITIONING FOR ABDOMINAL SONOGRAPHY

- Most often, abdominal sonographic imaging is initially conducted in the supine position.
- Other patient positions may be utilized throughout the exam, including upright and decubitus positioning **(Fig. 1-15)**.
- Decubitus and upright positions should be utilized in order to assess the mobility of intraluminal objects such as the presence of suspected gallstones or urinary bladder masses.

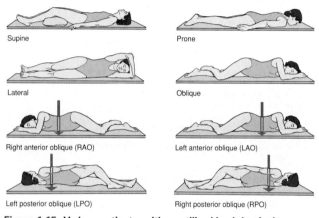

Supine

Prone

Lateral

Oblique

Right anterior oblique (RAO)

Left anterior oblique (LAO)

Left posterior oblique (LPO)

Right posterior oblique (RPO)

Figure 1-15. Various patient positions utilized in abdominal imaging. The upright position is not depicted here. (Reprinted with permission from Penny SM, ed. *Introduction to Sonography and Patient Care*. Philadelphia, PA: Wolters Kluwer; 2015.)

LABELING OF SONOGRAPHIC EXAMINATIONS

- It is optimal to label the sonographic image with the scan plane utilized and the organ or structure being assessed.
- If another position other than supine is utilized during the examination, then providing the altered patient position is most advantageous for the interpreting physician.
- Accompanying digital arrows or specific text identifying organs, pathology, or structures can be beneficial for interpretation.
- Some organs, such as the breast, may have specific labeling requirements (e.g., clock face or quadrant) per institutional guidelines.
- Short videos or cine clips can provide insight into the relationship of organs, pathology, and structures. Specific labeling (e.g., medial-to-lateral or superior-to-inferior) may be required.

COMPLETE ABDOMEN AND RIGHT UPPER QUADRANT SUGGESTED PROTOCOL

- Complete abdominal sonogram protocol
  - The assessment can be performed in the following manner with patient in the supine position initially:
    - Pancreas*
    - Liver
    - Gallbladder and biliary tree
    - Right kidney
    - Aorta and IVC
    - Spleen
    - Left kidney
    - Decubitus examination of the gallbladder and biliary tree
  - When abnormalities, such as hydronephrosis, are suspected, the urinary bladder and pelvis should be assessed for associated pathology.
  - Upright imaging of the pancreas may be helpful if supine imaging is not accommodating.
  - Upright and prone imaging of the gallbladder may be helpful as well.
  - Focal areas of pain should be assessed as well.

---

*Some institutions may request initiating the examination with an analysis of the aorta and inferior vena cava.

- Right upper quadrant protocol
  - The assessment can be performed in the following manner with patient in the supine position initially:
    - Pancreas
    - Liver
    - Gallbladder and biliary tree
    - Right kidney
    - Decubitus examination of the gallbladder and biliary tree
  - When abnormalities, such as hydronephrosis, are suspected, the left kidney, urinary bladder, and pelvis should be assessed for associated pathology.
  - Upright imaging of the pancreas may be helpful if supine imaging is not accommodating.
  - Upright and prone imaging of the gallbladder may be helpful as well.
  - Focal areas of pain should be assessed as well.

FLUID RECOGNITION

- Chest
  - Pleural effusions may be visualized with sonography during an abdominal sonogram and should be documented (**Fig. 1-16**).
- Peritoneal cavity
  - The abdomen has several locations that are common abdominal fluid collection points, also referred to as ascites.
    - Right subhepatic space (**Fig. 1-17**)
      - ○ Also referred to as Morison pouch.
      - ○ Located between the right lobe of the liver and the right kidney.
      - ○ A common place for ascites to collect in the right upper quadrant.
    - Lesser sac
      - ○ Located between the pancreas and the stomach.
      - ○ A common location for a pancreatic pseudocyst to be located.
    - Subphrenic spaces
      - ○ Located inferior to the diaphragm.

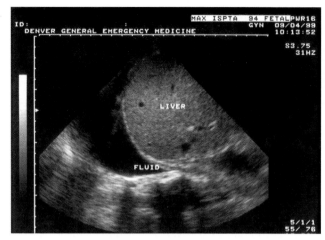

Figure 1-16. Pleural effusion. In this longitudinal image, fluid is noted superior to the liver and diaphragm, which is consistent with a right pleural effusion. (Image reprinted with permission from Cosby K, Kendall J, eds. *Practical Guide to Emergency Ultrasound*. Philadelphia, PA: Lippincott Williams & Wilkins; 2006:72.)

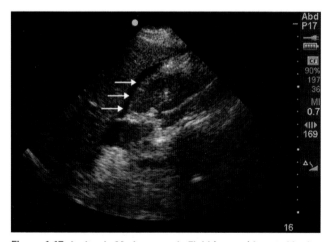

Figure 1-17. Ascites in Morison pouch. Fluid (*arrows*) is noted in the right subhepatic space, which is also referred to as Morison pouch. (Reprinted with permission from Bachur RG, Shaw KN, eds. *Fleisher and Ludwig's Textbook of Pediatric Emergency Medicine*. 7th ed. Philadelphia, PA: Wolters Kluwer; 2015.)

- Paracolic gutters
  - Bilateral gutters extend along the lateral margin of the peritoneum.
- Posterior cul-de-sac
  - In females, this space is located between the uterus and rectum.
  - It is also referred to as the rectouterine pouch or pouch of Douglas.
  - It is the most common place for fluid to collect in the pelvis.
- Anterior cul-de-sac
  - Space located between the urinary bladder and uterus.
  - Also referred to as the vesicouterine pouch.
- If ascites is identified in the right upper quadrant, an overall assessment of the other abdominal quadrants may be warranted to assess the general amount of ascites present.

FOCUSED ASSESSMENT WITH SONOGRAPHY FOR TRAUMA EXAMINATION[5]

- Sonography can be used to provide a quick analysis of the abdomen for evidence of intraperitoneal fluid.
- The FAST examination is used to evaluate the torso for bleeding after traumatic injury, particularly blunt trauma.
- See the training guidelines of the physician provider's specialty society regarding training and qualifications to perform the FAST exam.
- If appropriately trained, physician extenders, emergency medical personnel, and sonographers can obtain the sonographic images.
- Acute hemorrhage initially appears as an anechoic fluid collection. However, as blood clots, often rapidly, these fluid collections may appear complex, hypoechoic, or even isoechoic to surrounding structures.
- Common windows for assessment include (Fig. 1-18):
  - Right upper quadrant view
    - Includes an assessment of the right subhepatic space (Morison pouch), right pleural space, subphrenic spaces, and right paracolic gutter.

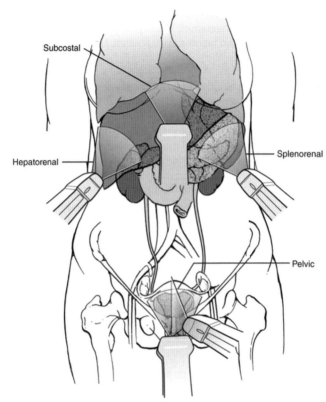

Figure 1-18. Common FAST exam transducer placement locations. Four sites of focused assessment of sonography for trauma (FAST) examination: subcostal, hepatorenal, splenorenal, and pelvic.
(Reprinted with permission from Berg SM, Bittner EA, Zhao KH, eds. *Anesthesia Review: Blasting the Boards.* Philadelphia, PA: Wolters Kluwer; 2016.)

- Left upper quadrant view
  - Includes an assessment of the perisplenic space above the spleen and below the diaphragm, left pleural space, and left paracolic gutter.
- Pelvic view
  - Includes evaluation of the pelvic spaces, including the anterior and posterior culs-de-sac.
- Pericardial view
  - Includes subcostal images of the sagittal and transverse four-chamber views of the heart, pericardial space, and an analysis of the inferior vena cava and hepatic veins.
- Anterior thoracic view
  - Includes an analysis of the lung pleura for the normal sliding typically noted. This is most often imaged in the second or third intercostal space with a higher frequency transducer because of the superficial imaging required.
  - An assessment for pneumothorax is provided by evaluating for signs of a lung point, which represents the site where the lung adheres to the parietal pleura immediately adjacent to the pneumothorax.
- Other supplementary views may be utilized, including inferior vena cava views, right and left paracolic gutter views, pleural space views, parasternal views, and apical views.

INFECTION CONTROL AND MACHINE MAINTENANCE

- Transducers and transducer cords should be cleaned with an appropriate disinfectant solution or wiped according to the manufacturers' recommendations. The ultrasound machine keyboard and surfaces should be routinely cleaned as well.
- Stretchers should also be cleaned before and after each patient.
- A scheduled preventative maintenance plan for all ultrasound equipment should be established based on the manufacturers' recommendations to ensure that diagnostic quality images are maintained and patient safety is optimized.

ERGONOMICS[2]

- Ergonomics is the scientific study of creating tools and equipment that help humans adapt to the work environment.

- Proper ergonomics in sonographic practice includes the use of proper room design and appropriately adjustable equipment.
- Sonographers should utilize equipment that minimizes the likelihood of developing a work-related musculoskeletal disorder.
- Best practices include the following:
  - Minimize sustained bending, twisting, reaching, lifting, pressure, and awkward postures.
  - Place the patient as close to you as possible to reduce reaching and shoulder abduction.
  - Use correct body mechanics when moving patients.
  - Relax muscles periodically throughout the day.
  - Position equipment to reduce awkward postures and promote neck, back, shoulder, and arm comfort.
  - If pain manifests, take a short break, and change your position immediately.

REFERENCES

1. AIUM practice parameters for the performance of an ultrasound of the abdomen and/or retroperitoneum. http://www.aium.org/resources/guidelines/abdominal.pdf. Accessed November 24, 2018.
2. Penny SM. *Introduction to Sonography and Patient Care*. Philadelphia, PA: Wolters Kluwer; 2016:58.
3. Sander RC, Hall-Terracciano BH. *Clinical Sonography: A Practical Guide*. 5th ed. Philadelphia, PA: Wolters Kluwer; 2016:21–38; 61–93.
4. Penny SM. *Examination Review for Ultrasound: Abdomen & Obstetrics and Gynecology*. 2nd ed. Philadelphia, PA: Wolters Kluwer; 2018:168–178.
5. AIUM practice parameter for the performance of the focused assessment with sonography for trauma (FAST) examination. https://www.aium.org/resources/guidelines/fast.pdf. Accessed November 24, 2018.

1. Abdominal Sonography

CHAPTER 2

Pancreas

INTRODUCTION

The pancreas is often a hurriedly abandoned abdominal organ because of the challenges that it presents to the sonographer in regards to visualizing the entire organ with sonography. Surrounding bowel gas and large body habitus often lead to limitations for ultrasound beam interrogation, which in turn produces subsequent frustration for the sonographer. Nonetheless, because the pancreas is a vital abdominal organ, the necessary time should be invested exhausting varying techniques—including upright imaging and decubitus positioning—in order to visualize its entire structure. The pancreas is infrequently exclusively imaged with sonography, and thus an assessment of the liver and biliary tree are typically performed as well. Thus, the pancreas is often routinely included in the sonographic assessment of the right upper quadrant and complete abdomen.

AIUM RECOMMENDATIONS FOR SONOGRAPHY OF THE PANCREAS[1]

- Assess the pancreas in the following manner:
  - The pancreas should be assessed for parenchymal abnormalities (e.g., masses, cysts, calcifications, etc.).
  - The distal common bile duct should be evaluated in the region of the pancreatic head.
  - The pancreatic duct should be assessed for dilatation, which can be confirmed by measurement.
  - The peripancreatic anatomy should be observed for abnormalities such as lymphadenopathy, pancreatic pseudocysts, and/or fluid.

ESSENTIAL ANATOMY AND PHYSIOLOGY OF THE PANCREAS[2,3]

- Sections of the pancreas include the head, uncinate process, neck, body, and tail (**Fig. 2-1**).
- The pancreas is located in the anterior retroperitoneum and epigastric region (traverses the midline), with the head positioned within the C-loop of the duodenum and tail resting medial to the splenic hilum.
- The head is typically more caudally located compared to the body and tail.
- The main pancreatic duct may be referred to as the duct of Wirsung.
- The main pancreatic duct merges with the common bile duct at the ampulla of Vater and empties digestive juices through the sphincter of Oddi, also referred to as the major duodenal papilla (**Fig. 2-2**).
- The pancreas is both an endocrine and exocrine gland.
  - The endocrine function of the pancreas is to produce glucagon, insulin, and somatostatin.
  - The exocrine function of the pancreas includes the production of the digestive enzymes amylase, lipase, sodium bicarbonate, trypsin, chymotrypsin, and carboxypolypeptidase.

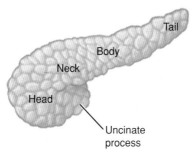

Figure 2-1. Basic pancreas anatomy. (Image reprinted with permission from Moore KL, Dalley AF II, Agur AMR, eds. *Clinically Oriented Anatomy.* 6th ed. Philadelphia, PA: Wolters Kluwer Health/Lippincott Williams & Wilkins; 2009.)

2. Pancreas

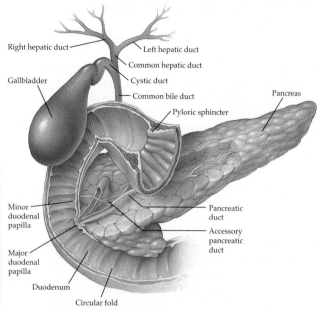

Figure 2-2. Anatomy of the pancreas and the biliary tree. (Reprinted with permission from Anatomical Chart Company. *Digestive System Anatomical Chart.* Philadelphia, PA: Lippincott Williams & Wilkins; 2000.)

- Surrounding vasculature (**Fig. 2-3**):
  - Pancreatic head—right lateral to the superior mesenteric vein, anterior to the inferior vena cava, inferior to the portal vein
  - Uncinate process—posterior to the superior mesenteric vein and anterior to the abdominal aorta
  - Pancreatic neck—anterior to the portal confluence
  - Pancreatic body—anterior to the superior mesenteric vein, splenic vein, and superior mesenteric artery
  - Pancreatic tail—anterior to the splenic vein

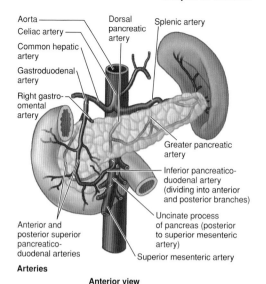

Aorta
Celiac artery
Common hepatic artery
Gastroduodenal artery
Right gastro-omental artery
Dorsal pancreatic artery
Splenic artery
Greater pancreatic artery
Inferior pancreatico-duodenal artery (dividing into anterior and posterior branches)
Uncinate process of pancreas (posterior to superior mesenteric artery)
Superior mesenteric artery
Anterior and posterior superior pancreatico-duodenal arteries

Arteries

Anterior view

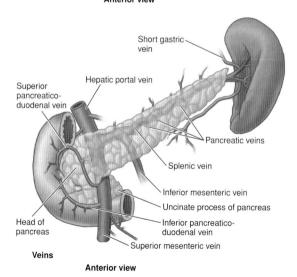

Short gastric vein
Hepatic portal vein
Superior pancreatico-duodenal vein
Pancreatic veins
Splenic vein
Inferior mesenteric vein
Uncinate process of pancreas
Inferior pancreatico-duodenal vein
Head of pancreas
Superior mesenteric vein

Veins

Anterior view

Figure 2-3. Surrounding vasculature of the pancreas. (Reprinted with permission from Moore KL, Dalley AF II, Agur AMR, eds. *Clinically Oriented Anatomy.* 7th ed. Philadelphia, PA: Wolters Kluwer Health/Lippincott Williams & Wilkins; 2013.)

2. Pancreas

PATIENT PREPARATION FOR SONOGRAPHY OF THE PANCREAS

- Patient preparation is focused on eliminating adjacent or overlying bowel gas that may inhibit sound beam penetration.
- NPO for 6–8 hrs is optimal, though fewer hours may be required, especially for pediatric cases or those requiring emergency sonographic investigation.

SUGGESTED EQUIPMENT

- 3–5-MHz transducer (higher frequencies can be used for thin patients and a large footprint transducer may be used to assist in the compression of the abdomen)
- General abdominal setting (most machines)
- Positional sponges for decubitus images

CLINICAL INVESTIGATION FOR SONOGRAPHY OF THE PANCREAS

- Laboratory values are listed in **Table 2-1.**[2,4]
- Evaluate prior imaging reports and images including CT, MRI, radiography, ERCP, and any other appropriate tests.
- Critical clinical history questions related to the pancreas:
  - History of pancreatitis? *The sonographic appearance of the pancreas may be altered in the presence of acute pancreatitis or chronic pancreatitis. Diffuse acute pancreatitis may appear as a hypoechoic, enlarged pancreas, while chronic pancreatitis leads to atrophy of the gland and it may contain calcifications and an enlarged main pancreatic duct.*
  - History of abdominal surgery (pancreatic surgery or cholecystectomy)? *A history of abdominal surgery of the pancreas, especially if part of the pancreas was removed, will alter the appearance of the pancreas sonographically.*
  - Epigastric or back pain? *Pancreatitis could result in epigastric and/or back pain.*
  - Nausea and/or vomiting? *Patients with pancreatitis could suffer from nausea and vomiting.*
  - History of gallstones? *Gallstones can lead to pancreatitis.*
  - Fever? *Patients with pancreatitis will often have a fever.*
  - Diabetic? *Diabetes may alter the echogenicity of the pancreas, often producing a diffusely hyperechoic appearance.*

Table 2-1	LAB FINDINGS AND POSSIBLE ASSOCIATED PANCREAS PATHOLOGY

LAB FINDING	POTENTIAL PANCREAS PATHOLOGY[2,4]
↑ Bilirubin and urobilirubin	Biliary obstruction, pancreatic disease, or possible liver disease
↑ Amylase	Acute pancreatitis, biliary or associated pancreatic obstruction, or other pancreatic disease such as pancreatic cancer
↑ Lipase	Acute pancreatitis, biliary or associated pancreatic obstruction, or other pancreatic disease such as pancreatic cancer
↑ ALT	Biliary tract disease or associated pancreatic disease
↑ ALP	Pancreatic disease such as chronic pancreatitis, cholelithiasis, biliary obstruction, or possible liver disease
↑ AST	Pancreatic disease or associated liver disease
↑ WBC	Pancreatitis, cholecystitis, cholangitis, or other inflammatory diseases/infection

- Unexplained weight loss? *Patients with pancreatic cancer or chronic pancreatitis may suffer from unexplained weight loss.*

NORMAL SONOGRAPHIC DESCRIPTION OF THE PANCREAS

- The normal pancreas is said to be hyperechoic to the liver, though it may be isoechoic or even hypoechoic in patients with minimal body fat. Nonetheless, careful clinical assessment should be completed when an enlarged, hypoechoic pancreas is visualized, as this may represent sonographic signs of acute pancreatitis.
- A hyperechoic pancreas may represent fatty infiltration of the pancreas.
- In the head of the pancreas, there may be two anechoic circular structures.
  - The anterior structure is most likely the gastroduodenal artery.

- The posterior structure is most likely the common bile duct.
- The main pancreatic duct may appear as a linear tubular structure traversing the pancreatic body.
- In transverse, the anechoic vasculature structure of the portal splenic confluence and splenic vein should be seen marking the posterior borders of the pancreas.

SUGGESTED PROTOCOL FOR SONOGRAPHY OF THE PANCREAS

- Survey the pancreas in transverse
  - With the patient in the supine position, obtain a brief survey of the pancreas by scanning superiorly and inferiorly through the pancreas completely.
  - Perform a brief cine clip (**Video 2-1**).
- Transverse pancreas (demonstrate head, neck, body) (**Fig. 2-4**)
  - Place the transducer in the midline of the body in the epigastrium, just below the xyphoid process of the sternum (**Fig. 2-5**).
  - Using the left lobe of the liver, angle slightly inferior to visualize the head, neck, and body of the pancreas.
    - The transducer may be slightly tilted or angled to the patient's right side and inferiorly to see the pancreatic head.
    - Helpful vascular landmarks include the portal splenic confluence and superior mesenteric vein, which are located posterior to the neck of the pancreas. The splenic vein is located posterior to the body (**Fig. 2-6**).
    - Two, round anechoic structures may be seen in the head of the pancreas, the most anterior structure is most likely the gastroduodenal artery, and the most posterior structure is most likely the distal common bile duct (**Fig. 2-7**).
  - Analyze the borders of the pancreas and its echogenicity.
    - The normal pancreas should be uniform in echogenicity.
  - Assess the pancreas for possible dilatation of the pancreatic duct.
  - Evaluate the pancreas for solid masses, ductal stones, calcifications, and cystic lesions.

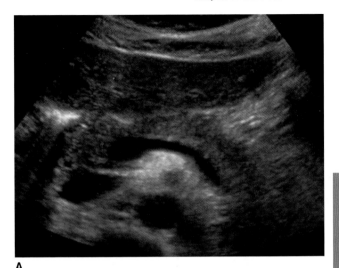

A

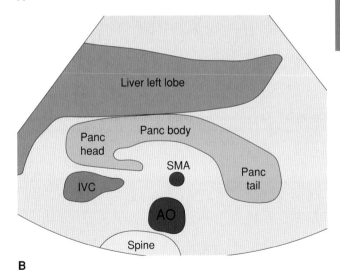

B

Figure 2-4. Transverse pancreas. A,B: Pancreas in the transverse plane demonstrating the *left lobe* of the liver, the pancreatic head (*Panc Head*), the pancreatic body (*Panc Body*), the pancreatic tail (*Panc Tail*), the superior mesenteric artery (*SMA*), the inferior vena cava (*IVC*), the abdominal aorta (*AO*), and the *spine*.

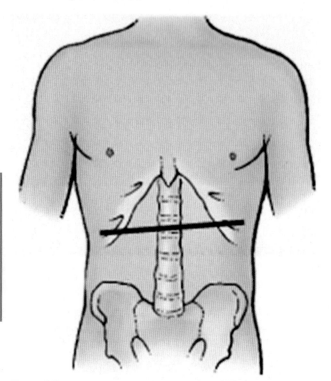

Figure 2-5. Correct scanning plane to obtain a transverse pancreas.
(Reprinted with permission from Agur AMR, Dalley AF, eds. *Grant's Atlas of Anatomy.* 14th ed. Philadelphia, PA: Wolters Kluwer; 2016.)

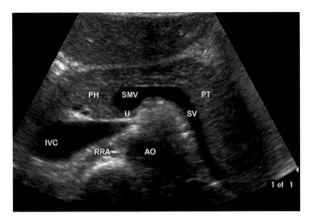

Figure 2-6. Transverse sonogram of the pancreas demonstrating adjacent vasculature. The pancreatic head (PH) is noted right lateral to the superior mesenteric vein (SMV). The splenic vein (SV) can be seen outlining the posterior aspect of the pancreatic tail (PT). AO, aorta; IVC, inferior vena cava; RRA, right renal artery; U, uncinate process. (Image courtesy of Philips Medical Systems, Bothell, WA.)

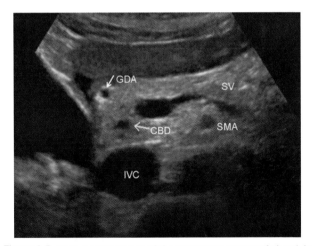

Figure 2-7. Sonographic image of the transverse pancreatic head. In this image, the gastroduodenal artery (*GDA*) and common bile duct (*CBD*) are noted within the head of the pancreas. IVC, inferior vena cava; SMA, superior mesenteric artery; SV, splenic vein. (Reprinted with permission from Kawamura D, Nolan T, eds. *Abdomen and Superficial Structures.* 4th ed. Philadelphia, PA: Wolters Kluwer; 2017.)

- If required, measure the head and body of the pancreas
  (Figs. 2-8 and 2-9).
- Transverse pancreas (demonstrates tail)
  - Slightly tilt or angle the transducer to the patient's left side
    and inferiorly to see the pancreatic tail.
    - The splenic vein is located posterior to the body and tail
      of the pancreas.
  - If required, measure the tail of the pancreas **(Fig. 2-10).**
- Longitudinal pancreas **(Fig. 2-11)**
  - Place the transducer just right of the midline in the
    longitudinal plane, just below the xyphoid process, to
    obtain a longitudinal image of the pancreas.
  - Note the head of the pancreas anterior to the IVC and
    inferior to the portal vein.
  - From the level of the head, scanning the left lateral, note
    the body left of the midline anterior to the aorta and
    superior mesenteric artery.
  - To visualize the tail, place the patient in the right lateral
    decubitus position. However, this may not be optimal (see
    Additional images section below).
- Additional images
  - Longitudinal or transverse right lateral decubitus
    pancreatic tail **(Fig. 2-12)**
    - The pancreatic tail rests medial to the splenic hilum.
    - The patient should be in the right lateral decubitus
      position. In longitudinal or transverse, scanning through
      the spleen, one can possibly visualize the pancreatic tail
      medial to the splenic hilum.
  - Transverse upright pancreas
    - Having the patient sit upright or stand can assist in the
      visualization of the pancreas occasionally.
    - Transducer placement is in the midline of the body in
      the epigastrium, just below the xyphoid process of the
      sternum. Somewhat lower transducer placement may be
      warranted with the patient in the upright position.

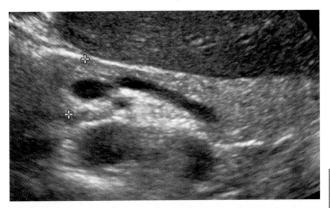

Figure 2-8. Pancreatic head measurement. In the transverse plane, a measurement of the pancreatic head (between *calipers*) can be obtained. (Reprinted with permission from Kawamura D, Nolan T, eds. *Abdomen and Superficial Structures*. 4th ed. Philadelphia, PA: Wolters Kluwer; 2017.)

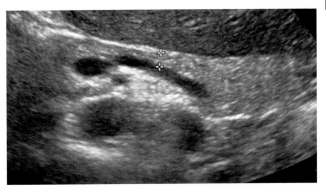

Figure 2-9. Pancreatic body measurement. In the transverse plane, a measurement of the pancreatic body (between *calipers*) can be obtained. (Reprinted with permission from Kawamura D, Nolan T, eds. *Abdomen and Superficial Structures*. 4th ed. Philadelphia, PA: Wolters Kluwer; 2017.)

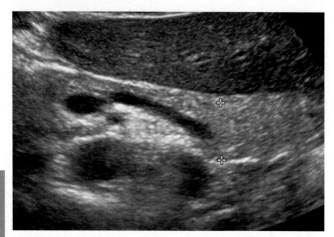

Figure 2-10. Pancreatic tail measurement. In the transverse plane, a measurement of the pancreatic tail (between *calipers*) can be obtained. (Reprinted with permission from Kawamura D, Nolan T, eds. *Abdomen and Superficial Structures.* 4th ed. Philadelphia, PA: Wolters Kluwer; 2017.)

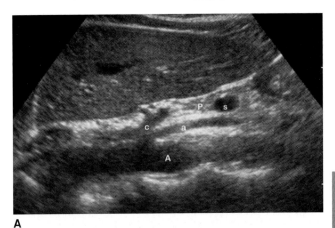

A

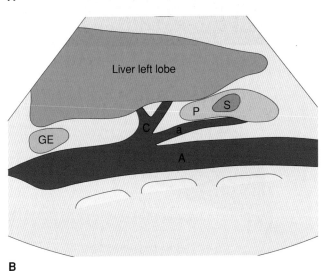

B

Figure 2-11. **Longitudinal pancreas. A,B: Longitudinal image of the pancreas demonstrating the left lobe of the liver, gastroesophageal junction (GE), celiac trunk (C), pancreas (P), splenic vein (S), abdominal aorta (A), and superior mesenteric artery.** (Reprinted with permission from Kawamura D, Nolan T, eds. *Abdomen and Superficial Structures.* 4th ed. Philadelphia, PA: Wolters Kluwer; 2017.)

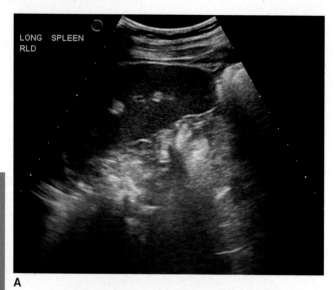

A

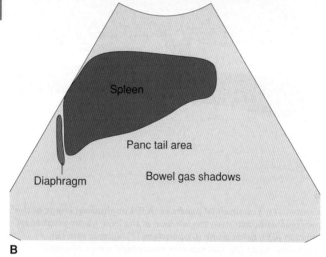

B

Figure 2-12. **Right lateral decubitus pancreas. A,B:** Longitudinal spleen in RLD demonstrating the splenic hilum and the area of the pancreatic tail.

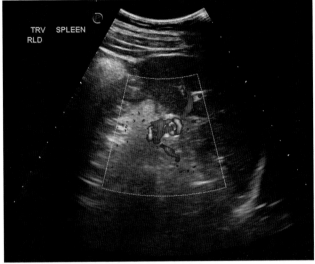

C

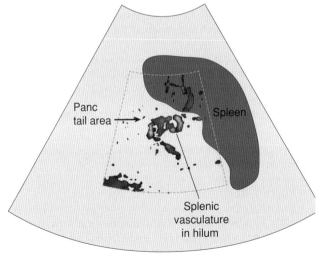

D

Figure 2-12 *(continued)*. C,D: Transverse spleen in RLD with color Doppler demonstrating the splenic hilum and the area of the pancreatic tail.

SCANNING TIPS

- Use the left lobe of the liver as an acoustic window.
- Use compression to displace bowel gas in the area of the pancreas.
- Ask the patient to completely exhale while scanning.
- Ask the patient to push his/her abdomen out or tighten abdominal muscles (Valsalva maneuver).
- Have the patient take in a deep breath and hold that breath while you scan.
- Once the exam is complete, utilize upright imaging over the area of the pancreas if the pancreas was not visualized.
- If not contraindicated, have the patient ingest a small amount of water. Water within the stomach and proximal duodenum can be used to provide an acoustic window to highlight the head and other sections of the pancreas.
- Try imaging the pancreas in various decubitus positions to better visualize all of its structure.
- Image the tail of the pancreas from the left lateral splenic window adjacent to the splenic hilum.
- If the patient has had or is currently suffering from pancreatitis, carefully analyze the lesser sac, which is located between the stomach and pancreas, for signs of a pancreatic pseudocyst.
- If the common bile duct appears enlarged in the head of the pancreas, attempt to follow the duct to the liver and evaluate the liver for signs of biliary dilatation as well.

NORMAL MEASUREMENTS OF THE PANCREAS[3,5,6]

- Male pancreas is on average larger than females.
- Anteroposterior dimension measurements are obtained in the true transverse plane.*
  - Head = 2–3.5 cm
  - Body = 2–3 cm
  - Tail = 1–2 cm
  - Main pancreatic duct = ~2 mm (may be up to 3.5 mm near the head, 2.5 mm in the body, and 1.5 mm in the tail) (Fig. 2-13)

---

*Both imaging and clinical assessment must be correlated when pancreatic size or duct diameter is suspiciously enlarged.

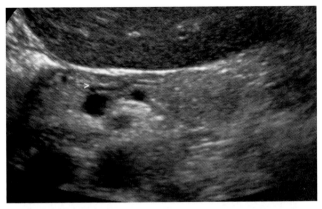

Figure 2-13. Transverse pancreas with pancreatic duct. The main pancreatic duct (*arrowhead*) is noted within the neck and body of this pancreas. (Reprinted with permission from Kawamura D, Nolan T, eds. *Abdomen and Superficial Structures.* 4th ed. Philadelphia, PA: Wolters Kluwer; 2017.)

ESSENTIAL PANCREATIC PATHOLOGY[2]

- Acute pancreatitis—inflammation of the pancreas **(Fig. 2-14)**
  - Clinical findings:
    - Elevated amylase, lipase, WBC, and ALT and other liver function tests
    - Decrease in hematocrit (with hemorrhagic pancreatitis)
    - Back pain or abdominal pain
    - Fever
    - Nausea and vomiting
  - Sonographic findings:
    - Pancreas may appear normal
    - Diffusely, enlarged hypoechoic pancreas
    - Focal pancreatitis may appear as a focal, hypoechoic enlargement
    - Peripancreatic fluid
    - Pancreatic pseudocyst (most likely in the lesser sac)
    - Biliary dilatation
    - Assess for splenic vein thrombosis and pseudoaneurysms of the splenic artery

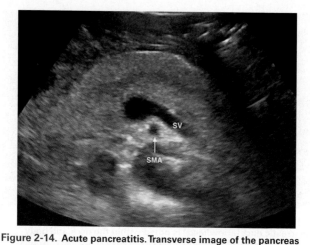

Figure 2-14. Acute pancreatitis. Transverse image of the pancreas in a patient with acute pancreatitis. The pancreas is edematous and enlarged. SMA, superior mesenteric artery; SV, splenic vein. (Reprinted with permission from Kawamura D, Nolan T, eds. *Abdomen and Superficial Structures*. 4th ed. Philadelphia, PA: Wolters Kluwer; 2017.)

- Chronic pancreatitis—chronic inflammation of the pancreas with atrophic changes **(Fig. 2-15)**
  - Clinical findings:
    - Possible elevation of amylase, lipase, and ALP
    - May be asymptomatic
    - Persistent epigastric pain
    - Jaundice
    - Back pain
    - Anorexia
    - Vomiting
    - Weight loss
    - Constipation
  - Sonographic findings:
    - Heterogeneous or hyperechoic gland
    - Poor margins with parenchymal calcifications
    - Pancreatic pseudocyst (most likely in the lesser sac)
    - Dilated pancreatic duct
    - Stones within the pancreatic duct
    - Assess for possible portosplenic vein thrombosis

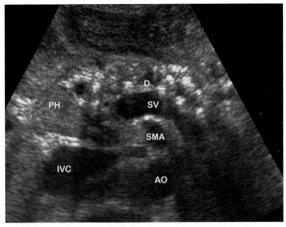

Figure 2-15. **Chronic pancreatitis. Transverse image of the pancreas in a patient with chronic pancreatitis. Calcifications are seen throughout the body and tail of the pancreas. AO, aorta; D, pancreatic duct; IVC, inferior vena cava; PH, pancreatic head; SMA, superior mesenteric artery; SV, splenic vein.** (Image courtesy of Philips Medical Systems, Bothell, WA.)

- Pancreatic carcinoma—most likely in the head of the pancreas **(Fig. 2-16)**
  - Clinical findings:
    - Elevated amylase, lipase, ALP, and other liver function tests
    - Weight loss
    - Loss of appetite
    - Jaundice
    - Courvoisier gallbladder (enlarged palpable gallbladder)
    - Epigastric pain
  - Sonographic findings:
    - Hypoechoic mass in the head of the pancreas (some cancerous tumors may have cystic components)
    - Dilated common bile duct proximal to the mass
    - Dilated pancreatic duct
    - Enlarged gallbladder
    - Assess the liver and other abdominal organs carefully for signs of metastasis

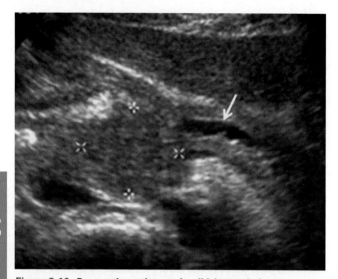

Figure 2-16. Pancreatic carcinoma. A solid, hypoechoic mass (between *calipers*) is noted within the head of the pancreas with associated dilation of the pancreatic duct (*arrow*). (Image reprinted with permission from Siegel MJ, ed. *Pediatric Sonography*. 4th ed. Philadelphia, PA: Wolters Kluwer Health/Lippincott Williams & Wilkins; 2010.)

WHERE ELSE TO LOOK

- Evaluate the entire biliary tree if pancreatic duct dilatation is suspected for further enlargement, stones, or other signs of obstruction.
- For patients with known pancreatitis, search the abdomen carefully for signs of a pancreatic pseudocyst. This cyst may appear mostly cystic but may have solid components as well.

IMAGE CORRELATION

- Normal pancreas on CT and MRI **(Fig. 2-17)**
- Acute pancreatitis on CT **(Fig. 2-18)**
- Chronic pancreatitis on CT **(Fig. 2-19)**

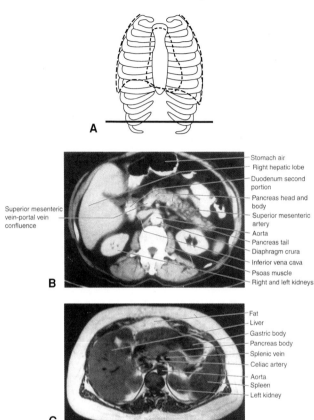

Figure 2-17. **The normal pancreas on CT and MRI. A: Illustration of the approximate axial anatomic level through the pancreas for B and C. B: Abdomen axial CT image through the pancreas level. C: Abdomen axial MR image through the pancreas level.** (Reprinted with permission from Erkonen WE, Smith WL, eds. *Radiology 101*. 3rd ed. Philadelphia, PA: Wolters Kluwer Health/Lippincott Williams & Wilkins; 2009.)

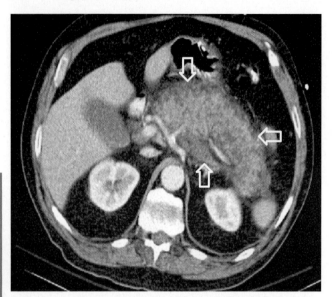

Figure 2-18. Acute pancreatitis on CT. An enlarged pancreas (between *arrows*) is noted in this CT of the abdomen, which is consistent with acute pancreatitis. (Reprinted with permission from Mulholland MW, Lillemoe KD, Doherty GM, Maier RV, Upchurch GR, eds. *Greenfield's Surgery*. 4th ed. Philadelphia, PA: Lippincott Williams & Wilkins; 2005.)

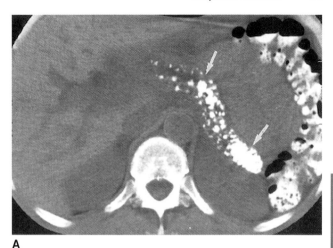

A

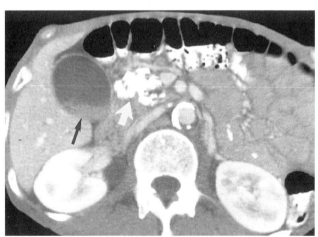

B

Figure 2-19. **Chronic pancreatitis on CT. A:** Unenhanced CT image through the pancreatic body reveals extensive coarse calcifications throughout the pancreas (*white arrows*). **B:** In the same patient, this enhanced CT image at the head of the pancreas shows coarse calcifications in the head (*white arrow*). There is also sludge in the dependent portion of the distended gallbladder (*black arrow*).

(Reprinted with permission from Pope TL Jr, Harris JH Jr, eds. *Harris & Harris' The Radiology of Emergency Medicine.* 5th ed. Philadelphia, PA: Wolters Kluwer Health/Lippincott Williams & Wilkins; 2012.)

REFERENCES

1. AIUM practice parameters for the performance of an ultrasound of the abdomen and/or retroperitoneum. http://www.aium.org/resources/guidelines/abdominal.pdf. Accessed June 27, 2018.
2. Penny SM. *Examination Review for Ultrasound: Abdomen & Obstetrics and Gynecology*. 2nd ed. Philadelphia, PA: Wolters Kluwer; 2018:1–78.
3. Kawamura DM, Nolan TD. *Diagnostic Medical Sonography: Abdomen and Superficial Structures*. 4th ed. Philadelphia, PA: Wolters Kluwer; 2018: 171–212.
4. Hopkins TB. *Lab Notes: Guide to Lab and Diagnostic Tests*. 2nd ed. Philadelphia, PA: F.A. Davis Company; 2009.
5. Curry RA, Tempkin BB. *Sonography: Introduction to Normal Structure and Function*. 4th ed. St. Louis, MO: Elsevier; 2016.
6. Rumack CM, Wilson SR, Charboneau JW, et al. *Diagnostic Ultrasound*. 4th ed. St. Louis, MO: Elsevier; 2011.

CHAPTER 3

Liver

INTRODUCTION

Though occasionally evaluated solitarily, the liver is often included with the sonographic analysis of the entire right upper quadrant or abdomen. When the liver is indeed solitarily examined, it is most often done so following other imaging studies, such as computed tomography scan as a follow-up procedure. Consequently, it is important most often to examine the surrounding structures in concert with the liver, including the abdominal aorta, inferior vena cava (IVC), gallbladder, biliary ducts, right kidney, and pancreas.

AIUM RECOMMENDATIONS FOR SONOGRAPHY OF THE LIVER[1]

- Assess the liver in the following manner:
  - Investigate each hepatic lobe (right, left, and caudate), and if possible, the right hemidiaphragm and the adjacent pleural space.
  - Evaluate the liver parenchyma for focal and diffuse abnormalities.
  - Compare the liver echogenicity with the echogenicity of the right kidney.
  - Evaluate the major hepatic and perihepatic vessels, including the IVC, the hepatic vein, the main portal vein, and if possible, the right and left portal vein.
  - Image the liver surface with a high-frequency transducer to assess for signs of surface nodularity in patients who may have cirrhosis.
  - For vascular examinations, use Doppler evaluation to document blood flow characteristics and the blood flow

direction. The structures that may be examined include the main and intrahepatic arteries, the hepatic veins, the main and intrahepatic portal veins, intrahepatic portion of the IVC, collateral venous pathways, and transjugular intrahepatic portosystemic shunt (TIPS) stents.

- Use elastography in patients who are predisposed to having hepatic fibrosis.

ESSENTIAL ANATOMY AND PHYSIOLOGY OF THE LIVER

- The liver is the largest parenchymal organ in the body, and it takes up most of the right upper quadrant and extends to the midline. In some individuals, the liver may come in contact with the spleen.
- The liver has three main lobes: right, left, and caudate.
  - The right and left lobes are separated by the middle hepatic vein, main lobar fissure, and gallbladder fossa.
  - Right lobe:
    - Located mostly on the right side of the abdomen.
    - Separated into anterior and posterior segments by the right hepatic vein.
  - Left lobe:
    - Located mostly in the midline.
    - Separated into medial and lateral segments by the left hepatic vein.
  - Caudate lobe:
    - Located in the midline, posterior to the left lobe.
    - Bordered anteriorly by the ligamentum venosum and posteriorly by the IVC.
  - The liver can be divided into eight surgical sections as well **(Fig. 3-1)**.
- The porta hepatis, also referred to as the liver hilum, is the area of the liver where the main portal vein and hepatic artery enter the liver and common bile duct exits the liver **(Fig. 3-2)**.
- The main portal vein is created from the union of the superior mesenteric vein and splenic vein.
  - The main portal vein enters the liver, bringing blood from the mesentery and other organs, and branches into right and left portal veins.

- The left portal vein branches into medial and lateral tributaries.
- The right portal vein branches into anterior and posterior tributaries.
- The right, middle, and left hepatic veins drain into the IVC **(Fig. 3-3)**.
- The hepatic artery is a branch of the celiac trunk.
- The liver performs many vital functions in order to maintain homeostasis including but not limited to:
  - Blood reservoir
  - Removal of waste products and detoxification
  - Vitamin and mineral storage
  - Creation of bile
  - Carbohydrate, fat, and amino acid metabolism

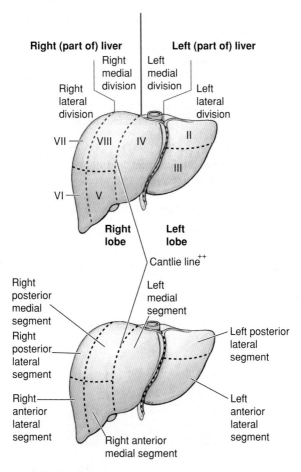

**Anterior views
(Diaphragmatic surface)**

**Figure 3-1. Parts, divisions, and segments of liver. Each part,
division, and segment has an identifying name; segments are
also identified by Roman numerals.** (Reprinted with permission from
Moore KL, Dalley AF, Agur AM, eds. *Clinically Oriented Anatomy.* 7th ed.
Philadelphia, PA: Wolters Kluwer Health/Lippincott Williams & Wilkins; 2013.)

3. Liver

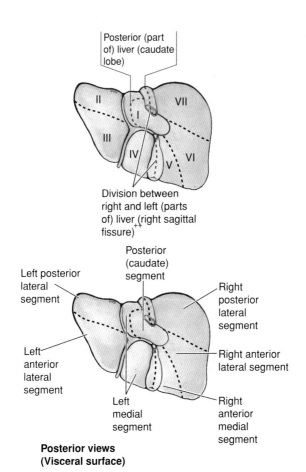

**Posterior views
(Visceral surface)**

Figure 3-1 *(continued)*.

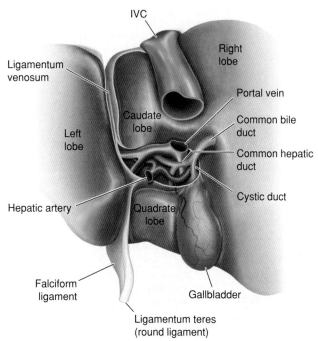

Figure 3-2. Drawing of the porta hepatis and surrounding structures. (Reprinted with permission from Kawamura D, Nolan T, eds. *Abdomen and Superficial Structures*. 4th ed. Philadelphia, PA: Wolters Kluwer; 2017.)

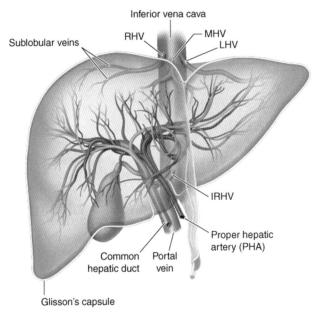

Figure 3-3. Vascular anatomy of the liver, including the portal vein, hepatic veins, and hepatic artery. (Reprinted with permission from Kawamura D, Nolan T, eds. *Abdomen and Superficial Structures.* 4th ed. Philadelphia, PA: Wolters Kluwer; 2017.)

PATIENT PREPARATION

- Patient preparation is focused on eliminating bowel gas and having the potential of a fully distended gallbladder at the time of the examination.
- NPO for 6–8 hrs is optimal, though fewer hours may be required, especially for pediatric cases or those requiring emergency sonographic investigation.
- If the examination is performed without fasting, proper documentation should take place.

SUGGESTED EQUIPMENT[1]

- 3–5-MHz transducer (higher frequencies can be used for thin patients)

3. Liver

- A high-frequency linear transducer to evaluate the contour of the liver for signs of nodular irregularity, especially in patients who have abnormal liver function
- General abdominal setting (most machines)
- Harmonics or supplementary artifact removal technology to eliminate false echoes
- Positional sponges for decubitus images

CLINICAL INVESTIGATION

- Laboratory values are listed in **Table 3-1**.[2]
- Evaluate prior imaging reports and images including CT, MRI, radiography, and any other appropriate tests.

Table 3-1	LABORATORY VALUES ASSOCIATED WITH LIVER FUNCTION AND POSSIBLE PATHOLOGIES[2]
LAB FINDINGS	**POTENTIAL PATHOLOGY**
↑ Alanine aminotransferase (ALT)	Biliary obstruction, hepatitis, hepatocellular disease, obstructive jaundice
↑ Alkaline phosphatase (ALP)	Cirrhosis, extrahepatic biliary obstruction, gallstones, hepatitis, liver cancer, pancreatic cancer
↑ Aspartate aminotransferase (AST)	Cirrhosis, fatty liver, hepatitis, liver metastasis
↑ Gamma-glutamyltransferase (GGT)	Diffuse liver disease and posthepatic obstruction
↑ Lactate dehydrogenase (LDH)	Cirrhosis, hepatitis, obstructive jaundice
↑ Serum bilirubin	Biliary obstruction, acute hepatocellular disease, cirrhosis, hepatitis, other liver cell diseases
↓ Albumin	Chronic liver disease and cirrhosis
Prothrombin time (PT)	Prolonged = liver metastasis or hepatitis Shortened = extrahepatic duct obstruction
↑ Alpha-fetoprotein (AFP)	Liver carcinoma

- Critical clinical history questions:
  - History of nausea and/or vomiting? *Patients with biliary-associated complaints often have nausea and/or vomiting.*
  - History of right upper quadrant pain? *If so, inquire about the length of time and the exact location of the pain if possible.*
  - History of abdominal surgeries? *This is important because the patient may have had a cholecystectomy or other biliary or liver surgery.*
  - History of hepatitis? *The sonographic appearance of the liver may be altered with hepatitis.*
  - History of alcoholism or cirrhosis? *The liver should be thoroughly assessed when cirrhosis is suspected for signs of portal hypertension and other complications, including portal vein thrombosis. Patients with cirrhosis who have a TIPS should undergo a thorough Doppler analysis of the shunt and other hepatic vascular anatomy.*

NORMAL SONOGRAPHIC DESCRIPTION OF THE LIVER

- The liver should be homogeneous and slightly more echogenic than or equal to that of the right kidney.
- The liver is typically isoechoic or more hypoechoic to the normal spleen.
- The normal liver parenchyma is occasionally interrupted by anechoic vascular structures.

SUGGESTED PROTOCOL FOR SONOGRAPHY OF THE LIVER

- Survey the liver in transverse or longitudinal:
  - Ask the patient to extend his or her right arm up above his or her head in order to expand the intercostal spaces.
  - With the patient in the supine position, obtain a brief survey of the liver by scanning superiorly and inferiorly (transverse) or medially and laterally (longitudinal).
  - Perform a brief cine clip in longitudinal and transverse **(Video 3-1 and Video 3-2)**.
- Longitudinal liver:
  - Assess the left lobe in the midline of the body and provide images of the left lobe by scanning medially and laterally.

Scan toward the patient's left side completely to assess the entire left lobe (Fig. 3-4).

- Image the caudate lobe and hepatic section of the IVC in longitudinal.
- From the midline, if possible, angle laterally toward the patient's right side to demonstrate the parenchyma of the right lobe. Angle the transducer from the midline toward the patient's right side.
- Demonstrate the level of the falciform ligament and main lobar fissure (Fig. 3-5).
- Position the transducer on the patient's right side and assess the right lobe of the liver.
  - Provide a liver–kidney interface image (Fig. 3-6). Evaluate the echogenicity of the liver compared to the right kidney, assess for fluid in the right subhepatic space (Morrison pouch), and for signs of a right-sided pleural effusion.
  - Provide several images of the right lobe of the liver while scanning through the patient's provided sonographic windows by angling the transducer throughout the windows (Fig. 3-7).
- Transverse liver:
  - Assess the left lobe and caudate lobe in the midline of the body and provide images of the left lobe and caudate lobe by scanning superiorly and inferiorly (Fig. 3-8).
  - From the midline, if possible, angle superiorly and laterally toward the patient's right shoulder to demonstrate the parenchyma of the right lobe. Some obliquity of the transducer may be required.
    - Provide images of the hepatic veins and IVC (Fig. 3-9).
    - Provide images of the portal veins and their branches (Fig. 3-10).
  - Position the transducer on the patient's right side and assess the right lobe of the liver.
    - Provide several images of the right lobe of the liver, including the most superior and inferior aspects of the liver.

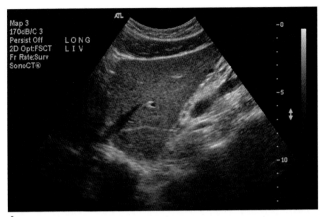

A

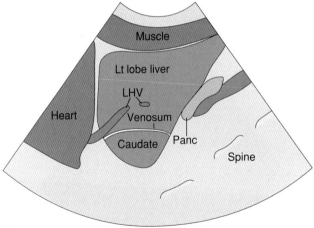

B

Figure 3-4. **Left lobe of the liver in longitudinal. A,B: Longitudinal left lobe (*Lt lobe liver*) and caudate lobe. This image also demonstrates the location of the ligamentum venosum (Venosum), pancreas (*Panc*), left hepatic vein (*LHV*), anterior musculature (*muscle*), heart, and spine.**

3. Liver

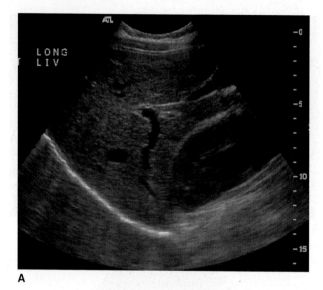

A

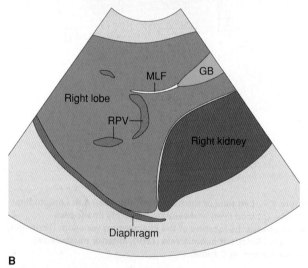

B

Figure 3-5. Longitudinal image of the main lobar fissure.
A,B: The main lobar fissure (*MLF*) is noted in this image of right lobe, gallbladder, and right portal vein (*RPV*). Also demonstrated is the right kidney and diaphragm.

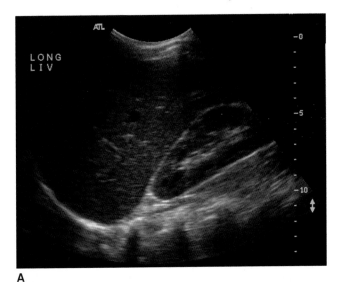

A

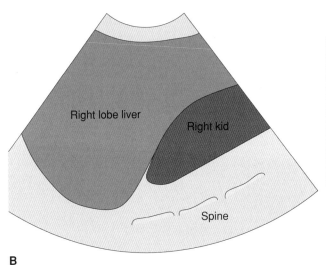

B

Figure 3-6. Liver–kidney interface. A,B: Image of the right lobe of the liver and the right kidney (*Right kid*) can be used to examine the echogenicities of the liver and the right kidney.

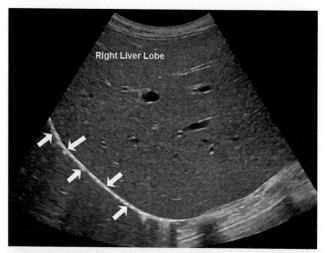

Figure 3-7. Longitudinal images of the right lobe. Normal sonographic image of the right lobe of the liver and the diaphragm.
(Reprinted with permission from Kawamura D, Lunsford B, eds. *Abdomen and Superficial Structures*. 3rd ed. Philadelphia, PA: Wolters Kluwer Health/ Lippincott Williams & Wilkins; 2012.)

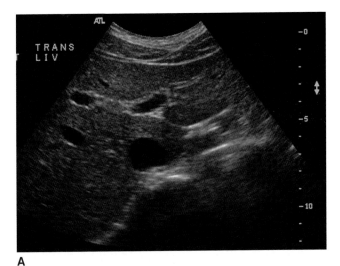

A

B

Figure 3-8. Transverse image of the left lobe. A,B: Transverse image of the left lobe (*LT lobe*) and caudate lobe (*Caudate*). The ligamentum venosum (*VEN*) can be seen separating the left lobe and caudate lobe, with inferior vena cava (*IVC*) posterior to the caudate. The left portal (*LT port*) and right lobe can also be seen (*RT lobe*).

3. Liver

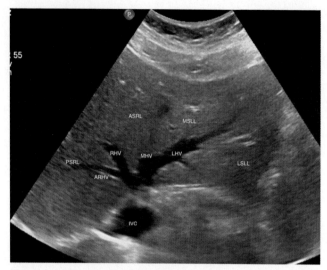

Figure 3-9. Transverse hepatic veins. A transverse section through the liver at the level of the hepatic veins. ASRL, anterior segment of the right lobe; **ARHV,** accessory right hepatic vein; **LSLL,** lateral segment left lobe; **LHV,** left hepatic vein; **MHV,** middle hepatic vein; **MSLL,** medial segment left lobe; **PSRL,** posterior segment of the right lobe; **RHV,** right hepatic vein. (Reprinted with permission from Kawamura D, Nolan T, eds. *Abdomen and Superficial Structures.* 4th ed. Philadelphia, PA: Wolters Kluwer; 2017.)

- Provide an image of the porta hepatis and branches of the portal veins if possible **(Fig. 3-11).**
- Provide several images of the right lobe of the liver while scanning through the patient's provided sonographic windows by angling the transducer throughout the windows.
  - Additional images:
    - Some institutions' sonographic protocols, such as a complete abdominal sonogram or right upper quadrant, include required images of the pancreas, gallbladder, bile ducts, and right kidney. Please see the associated chapters in this text for further guidance.
    - Doppler assessment of the hepatic vasculature:
      - Provide images that include Doppler interrogation of the main portal vein, hepatic artery, and

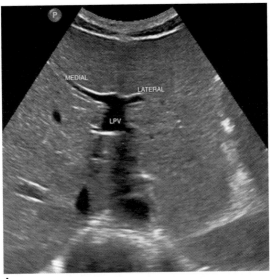

A

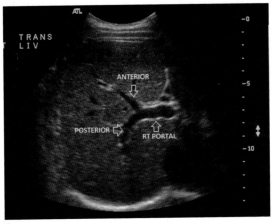

B

Figure 3-10. Transverse portal veins. A: Transverse image of the left portal vein (*LPV*) demonstrating its medial and lateral branches. B: Transverse image of the right portal vein (*RT PORTAL*) and its posterior and anterior branches. (Part A reprinted with permission from Kawamura D, Nolan T, eds. *Abdomen and Superficial Structures.* 4th ed. Philadelphia, PA: Wolters Kluwer; 2017.)

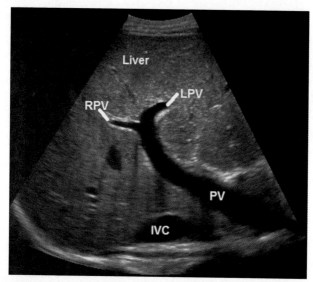

Figure 3-11. An oblique plane through the right upper quadrant visualizes the portal vein (*PV*) as it enters the liver and branches into the right portal vein (*RPV*) and the left portal vein (*LPV*). (Courtesy of Philips Medical System, Bothell, WA.)

hepatic veins to demonstrate normal flow patterns **(Fig. 3-12).**

- – Upon Doppler interrogation, the main portal vein should normally yield evidence of monophasic, hepatopetal flow (toward the liver). Respiration may alter flow patterns within the main portal vein and postprandial patterns may demonstrate an increase in portal vein flow.
- – With Doppler examination, the hepatic veins should demonstrate triphasic, hepatofugal flow (away from the liver).
- With Doppler examination, the hepatic artery should demonstrate low-resistance, hepatopetal flow.
- If requested, measure the right lobe of the liver according to your institutions protocol.
- Provide an image of the surface of the left lobe of the liver with a high-frequency linear transducer in patients with potential or suspected cirrhosis **(Fig. 3-13).**

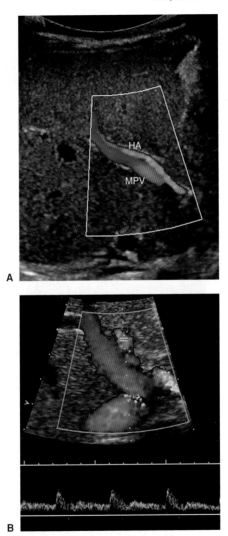

Figure 3-12. **Hepatic vasculature. A: Color Doppler of the hepatic artery. B: Color Doppler and spectral tracing of the normal hepatic artery.** *(continued)*

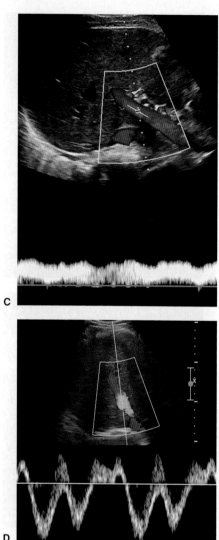

Figure 3-12 *(continued).* **C: Color Doppler and spectral of the normal main portal vein. D: Color Doppler and spectral of the normal middle hepatic vein.** (Reprinted with permission from Kawamura D, Nolan T, eds. *Abdomen and Superficial Structures.* 4th ed. Philadelphia, PA: Wolters Kluwer; 2017.)

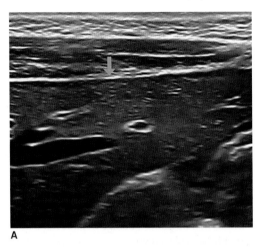

A

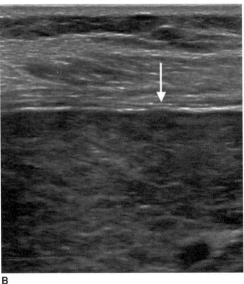

B

Figure 3-13. Sonogram of the liver surface with a linear transducer. A: An assessment of the surface of the liver should normally yield a smooth surface (*arrow*). B: A patient with cirrhosis often has a nodular appearing liver surface (*arrow*). (Reprinted with permission from Kawamura D, Nolan T, eds. *Abdomen and Superficial Structures*. 4th ed. Philadelphia, PA: Wolters Kluwer; 2017.)

3. Liver

SCANNING TIPS

- Deep, sustained inspiration can be helpful to assist in the visualization of the complete liver in most individuals.
- Some adjustment to sound penetration parameters may be required for patients who have a fatty liver or who are obese.
- Right lateral decubitus positioning can be helpful.

NORMAL MEASUREMENTS OF THE LIVER[3–5]

- Midhepatic or midclavicular line = <15 cm **(Fig. 3-14)**
- Enlargement of the liver may be visually suspected if the right lobe extends beyond the lower pole of the right kidney.

ESSENTIAL LIVER PATHOLOGY[2]

- Focal lesions:
  - Cavernous hemangioma—benign hepatic mass most commonly seen in women:
    - Clinical findings:
      ○ Asymptomatic
    - Sonographic findings:
      ○ Hyperechoic mass most often seen in the right lobe **(Fig. 3-15)**
  - Hepatic cysts:
    - Clinical findings:
      ○ Asymptomatic and may have normal liver function labs
      ○ May have a history of autosomal dominant polycystic kidney disease (ADPKD)
      ○ Hemorrhagic cysts or large cysts may cause pain and discomfort
    - Sonographic findings:
      ○ Anechoic mass with posterior enhancement **(Fig. 3-16)**
      ○ May have an irregular shape and may be multiple
- Diffuse liver disease:
  - Fatty liver (hepatic steatosis):
    - Clinical findings:
      ○ Asymptomatic
      ○ Alcohol abuse
      ○ Diabetes mellitus
      ○ Elevated liver function tests (AST and ALT)
      ○ Hyperlipidemia
      ○ Obesity
      ○ Pregnancy

3. Liver

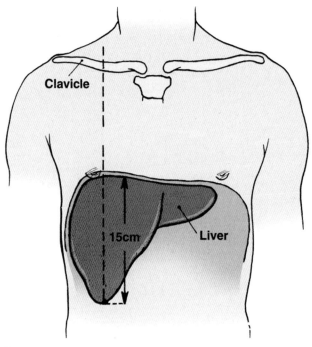

Figure 3-14. Measurement of the liver in the midclavicular line.
(Reprinted with permission from Sanders RC, ed. *Clinical Sonography: A Practical Guide.* 5th ed. Philadelphia, PA: Wolters Kluwer; 2015.)

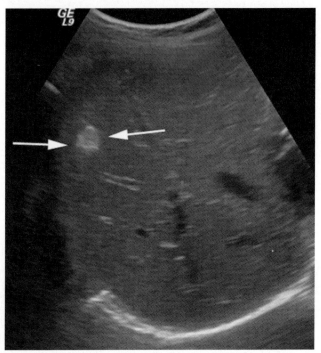

Figure 3-15. Cavernous hemangioma. This hyperechoic mass demonstrates the most common sonographic appearance of a cavernous hemangioma. (Reprinted with permission from Kawamura D, Nolan T, eds. *Abdomen and Superficial Structures*. 4th ed. Philadelphia, PA: Wolters Kluwer; 2017.)

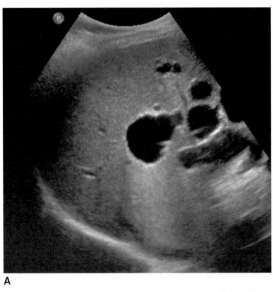

A

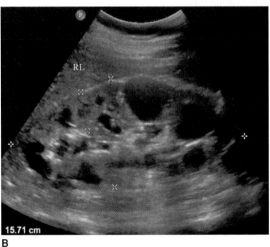

B

Figure 3-16. **Hepatic cysts. A: Hepatic cysts are noted as anechoic spaces within the liver. B: This patient also had renal cysts and was suffering from ADPKD.** (Reprinted with permission from Kawamura D, Lunsford B, eds. *Abdomen and Superficial Structures*. 3rd ed. Philadelphia, PA: Wolters Kluwer Health/Lippincott Williams & Wilkins; 2012.)

- Sonographic findings:
  - Diffusely echogenic liver (Fig. 3-17):
    - Fatty sparing—a hypoechoic area may be spared of fat and is often located adjacent to the gallbladder, porta hepatis, or an entire lobe may be spared
    - Focal infiltration—a hyperechoic focal area is demonstrated
  - Increased attenuation of the sound beam
  - Hepatic vasculature may be difficult to visualize
- Cirrhosis:
  - Clinical findings:
    - Ascites
    - Diarrhea
    - Elevated liver function tests
    - Fatigue
    - Initial hepatomegaly
    - Jaundice
    - Splenomegaly
    - Weight loss
  - Sonographic findings:
    - Initial hepatomegaly
    - Shrunken, echogenic right lobe (Fig. 3-18)
    - Enlarged caudate and left lobe
    - Nodular liver surface (noted best with a high-frequency linear transducer)
    - Splenomegaly
    - Ascites
    - Monophasic flow within the hepatic veins
    - Hepatofugal flow within the portal veins
- Hepatic metastasis:
  - Clinical findings:
    - Abnormal liver function tests
    - Weight loss
    - Jaundice
    - Right upper quadrant pain
    - Hepatomegaly
    - Abdominal swelling and ascites
  - Sonographic findings:
    - Hyperechoic, hypoechoic, calcified, cystic, or heterogeneous mass (Fig. 3-19)

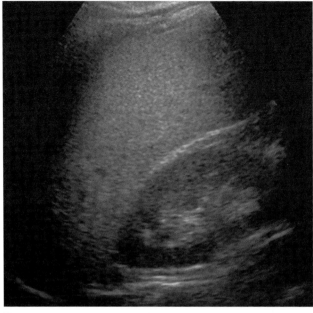

Figure 3-17. Fatty liver. Image of a fatty liver. Note the difficulty for sound beam penetration and lack of distinct border and vascularity. (Reprinted with permission from Kawamura D, Nolan T, eds. *Abdomen and Superficial Structures.* 4th ed. Philadelphia, PA: Wolters Kluwer; 2017.)

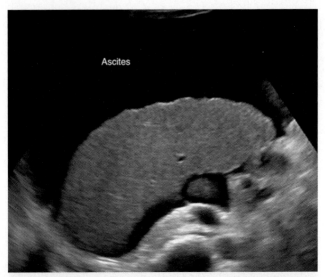

Figure 3-18. Cirrhotic liver. Image of a cirrhotic liver surrounded by ascites. (Reprinted with permission from Kawamura D, Nolan T, eds. *Abdomen and Superficial Structures*. 4th ed. Philadelphia, PA: Wolters Kluwer; 2017.)

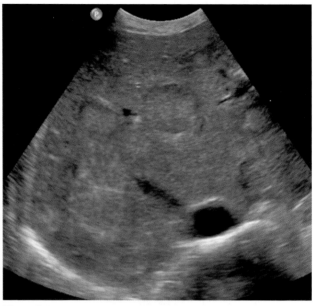

Figure 3-19. Liver metastasis. Multiple masses are visualized in this liver representing liver metastasis. (Reprinted with permission from Kawamura D, Lunsford B, eds. *Abdomen and Superficial Structures.* 3rd ed. Philadelphia, PA: Wolters Kluwer Health/Lippincott Williams & Wilkins; 2012.)

○ Mass with a notable hypoechoic rim and central echogenic portion
○ Diffusely heterogeneous liver
○ Possible ascites

WHERE ELSE TO LOOK

- Thoroughly evaluate the liver for signs of biliary obstruction. If noted, carefully evaluate the gallbladder and the pancreas for a recognizable cause for the obstruction.
- If cirrhosis is suspected, carefully evaluate the left portal vein for signs of recanalization of the paraumbilical vein, which is a sonographic sign of portal hypertension.
- If cirrhosis is suspected, evaluate the spleen for associated splenomegaly.
- If liver cysts are discovered, evaluate the kidneys carefully for associated cysts as well.

IMAGE CORRELATION

● CT and MRI of the liver (Figs. 3-20 and 3-21)

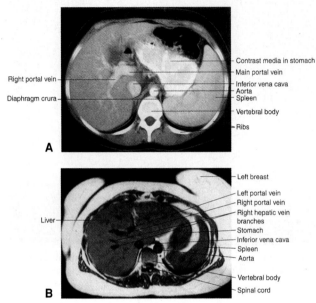

Figure 3-20. A: Abdomen axial CT image through the liver and spleen. B: Abdomen axial MR image through the liver and spleen. Normal. (Reprinted with permission from Erkonen WE, Smith WL, eds. *Radiology 101.* 3rd ed. Philadelphia, PA: Wolters Kluwer Health/Lippincott Williams & Wilkins; 2009.)

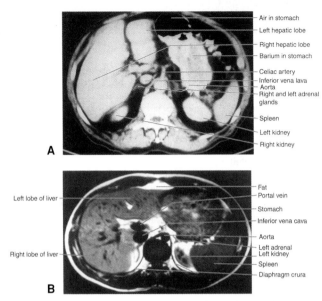

Figure 3-21. CT and MRI of the liver at the level of the right lobe. This level is just caudad to the level in Figure 3-20. A: Abdomen axial CT image through the liver and spleen. B: Abdomen axial MR image through the liver and spleen. (Reprinted with permission from Erkonen WE, Smith WL, eds. *Radiology 101*. 3rd ed. Philadelphia, PA: Wolters Kluwer Health/Lippincott Williams & Wilkins; 2009.)

REFERENCES

1. AIUM practice parameters for the performance of an ultrasound of the abdomen and/or retroperitoneum. http://www.aium.org/resources/guidelines/abdominal.pdf. Accessed September 19, 2018.
2. Penny SM. *Examination Review for Ultrasound: Abdomen & Obstetrics and Gynecology*. 2nd ed. Philadelphia, PA: Wolters Kluwer; 2018:1–67.
3. Rumack CM, Wilson SR, Charboneau JW, et al. *Diagnostic Ultrasound*. 4th ed. Philadelphia, PA: Elsevier; 2011:78–145.
4. Federle MF, Jeffrey RB Jr, Woodward PJ, Borhani A. *Diagnostic Imaging Abdomen*. 2nd ed. Altona, Manitoba, Canada: Amirsys; 2010:III:1:1–173.
5. Sanders RC, Hall-Terracciano B. *Clinical Sonography: A Practical Guide*. 5th ed. Philadelphia, PA: Wolters Kluwer; 2016:408–422.

CHAPTER 4

Gallbladder and Biliary Tract

INTRODUCTION

Sonography of the gallbladder is a common imaging examination. In fact, sonography is the gold standard for imaging of the gallbladder, and is especially utilized for patients with suspected cholelithiasis and accompanying cholecystitis. If achievable, varying patient position can assist in the identification of cholelithiasis. When gallbladder hydrops is present, especially accompanied by biliary dilatation, a thorough assessment of the entire biliary tract is warranted for the cause.

AIUM RECOMMENDATIONS FOR SONOGRAPHY OF THE GALLBLADDER AND BILIARY TRACT[1]

- Assess the gallbladder in the following manner:
  - The gallbladder should be distended, which will often require some time for fasting before the exam commences. Fasting time varies in regard to the age of the patient and overall physical condition.
  - The exam should include long-axis and transverse views of the gallbladder in the supine position and, in addition, decubitus imaging should be performed when feasible. Erect or prone imaging may be helpful as well.
  - A measurement of the gallbladder wall should be obtained.
- The patient should be assessed for the Murphy sign, which is tenderness to the transducer compression over the gallbladder (Fig. 4-1).
  - Assess the biliary tract in the following manner:
    - The intrahepatic ducts may be evaluated by obtaining views of the liver showing the right and left branches of the portal vein.

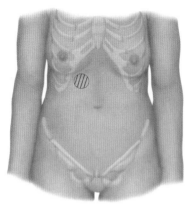

Figure 4-1. The Murphy sign. The Murphy sign is pain directly over the gallbladder elicited by transducer pressure. (Reprinted with permission from Bickley LS, Szilagyi P, eds. *Bates' Guide to Physical Examination and History Taking.* 8th ed. Philadelphia, PA: Lippincott Williams & Wilkins; 2003.)

- Color Doppler should be utilized in order to differentiate hepatic arteries and portal veins from bile ducts.
- The intrahepatic and extrahepatic bile ducts should be evaluated for dilatation, wall thickening, intraluminal findings, and other abnormalities.
- The bile duct in the area of the porta hepatis should be measured and documented.
- When visualized, the distal common bile duct in the pancreatic head should be evaluated.

ESSENTIAL ANATOMY AND PHYSIOLOGY OF THE GALLBLADDER AND BILIARY TRACT[2]

- Gallbladder (Fig. 4-2):
  - The cystic duct connects the gallbladder to the biliary tract.
  - The gallbladder has a partially inflated balloon shape that consists of a neck, body, and fundus.
  - The neck is the narrowest segment of the gallbladder and is thus the most common location for gallstones to become trapped.
  - The body is the widest segment of the gallbladder.
  - The fundus is the most dependent part of the gallbladder and is thus the most likely part to contain gallstones.

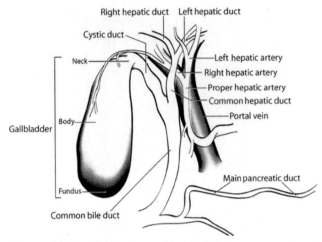

Figure 4-2. Detailed anatomy of the gallbladder. (Image reprinted with permission from Siegel MJ, ed. *Pediatric Sonography*. 4th ed. Philadelphia, PA: Wolters Kluwer Health/Lippincott Williams & Wilkins; 2010.)

- The gallbladder is used as a bile reservoir.
- When food reaches the duodenum, cholecystokinin is released by the cells of the duodenum, which causes the gallbladder to contract and partially empty itself of bile.
- Blood supply to the gallbladder is via the cystic artery, which is most likely a branch of the right hepatic artery.
- Bile ducts (see Fig. 4-2):
  - The biliary tract transports bile from the liver to the duodenum to be mixed with undigested foods.
  - Bile consists of cholesterol, bilirubin, biliverdin, and bile acids.
  - Exceedingly small biliary radicles, which are the most proximal segments of the biliary tract, are scattered throughout the liver parenchyma.
  - The biliary radicles eventually converge to form the right and left hepatic duct.
  - The right and left hepatic ducts join to form the common hepatic duct.
  - The cystic duct connects the gallbladder to the biliary tract and contains tiny structures that prevent collapse of the duct referred to as spiral valves of Heister.

- The common bile duct is the duct segment located distal to the cystic duct.
- The common bile duct joins the main pancreatic duct near the pancreatic head and the contents of pancreatic digestive juices and bile empty into the proximal duodenum.

PATIENT PREPARATION FOR SONOGRAPHY OF THE GALLBLADDER AND BILIARY TRACT[2,3]

- Patient preparation is focused on having the potential of a fully distended gallbladder at the time of the examination.
- NPO for 6–8 hrs is optimal, though fewer hours may be required, especially for pediatric cases or those requiring emergency sonographic investigation.
- If the examination is performed without fasting, proper documentation should take place.

SUGGESTED EQUIPMENT

- 3–5-MHz transducer (higher frequencies can be used for thin patients)
- General abdominal setting (most machines)
- Harmonics or supplementary artifact removal technology to eliminate false echoes
- Positional sponges for decubitus images

CLINICAL INVESTIGATION FOR SONOGRAPHY OF THE GALLBLADDER AND BILIARY TRACT

- Laboratory values are listed in **Table 4-1.**[2,4]
- Evaluate prior imaging reports and images including CT, MRI, radiography, ERCP, and any other appropriate tests.
- Critical clinical history questions:
  - History of cholecystectomy? **(Fig. 4-3)** *This is a vital question, especially if the gallbladder is not initially visualized in the right upper quadrant. Keep in mind that the common duct may be larger in patients who have had a cholecystectomy.*
  - History of right upper quadrant pain? *Patients with cholecystitis often have right upper quadrant pain.*
  - History of gallstones? *Some patients may know that they have been previously diagnosed with gallstones. Gallstones can lead to biliary obstruction and acute cholecystitis.*

Table 4-1	LAB FINDINGS AND POSSIBLE ASSOCIATED GALLBLADDER OR BILIARY TRACT PATHOLOGY
LAB FINDING	POTENTIAL GB/BILIARY TRACT PATHOLOGY[2,4]
↑ Bilirubin and urobilirubin	Biliary obstruction or possible liver or pancreatic disease
↑ Amylase	Biliary or associated pancreatic obstruction or other pancreatic disease
↑ Lipase	Biliary or associated pancreatic obstruction or other pancreatic disease
↑ ALT	Biliary tract disease or associated pancreatic disease
↑ ALP	Cholelithiasis or biliary obstruction and possible liver or pancreatic disease
↑ AST	Liver or pancreatic disease
↑ GGT	Liver disease, biliary obstruction, cholangitis
↑ WBC	Cholecystitis, cholangitis, or other inflammatory diseases/infection

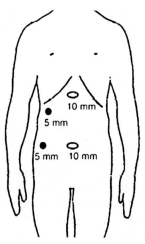

Figure 4-3. **Typical location of abdominal scars following a laparoscopic cholecystectomy. If the patient is unclear about past cholecystectomy and a gallbladder is not visualized, assess the patient for signs of abdominal scars in these locations.** (Modified with permission from Fischer J, ed. *Fischer's Mastery of Surgery.* 7th ed. Philadelphia, PA: Wolters Kluwer; 2018.)

- Postprandial right upper quadrant pain? *Right upper quadrant pain after eating a fatty meal may be a sign of acute cholecystitis.*
- Shoulder or chest pain? *Shoulder or chest pain can be a sign of acute cholecystitis.*
- Nausea and/or vomiting? *Patients with acute cholecystitis or biliary obstruction can suffer from nausea and vomiting.*
- History of liver or pancreatic disease? *Any previous history of liver or pancreatic disease should intensify sonographic scrutiny of the gallbladder and biliary tract.*

NORMAL SONOGRAPHIC DESCRIPTION OF THE GALLBLADDER AND BILIARY TRACT

- Gallbladder:
  - The gallbladder should be completely anechoic and typically has a balloon-shaped appearance.
  - The gallbladder wall should be thin (measuring <3 mm).
  - Folds may be present within the neck, body, or fundus.
- Bile ducts:
  - The intrahepatic ducts are not normally identifiable. If seen, the intrahepatic ducts appear as two parallel hyperechoic lines.
  - In longitudinal orientation to the porta hepatis, the common hepatic duct and common bile duct appear as tubular structures with an anechoic center.
  - In the transverse plane at the level of the pancreas, the distal common bile duct may be seen within the pancreatic head posterior to the gastroduodenal artery.

SUGGESTED PROTOCOL AND NORMAL ANATOMY OF THE GALLBLADDER AND BILIARY TRACT

- Gallbladder:
  - Survey the gallbladder:
    - The gallbladder fossa can be found by locating the main lobar fissure **(Fig. 4-4)**.
    - With the patient in the supine position, obtain a brief survey of the gallbladder in (either or both) the longitudinal and transverse scan planes.
    - A cine loop may be performed **(Video 4-1 and Video 4-2)**. 🎞

4. GB and Biliary

- Longitudinal gallbladder (Fig. 4-5):
  - Images should be oriented to the long axis of the gallbladder and thus the transducer may need to be placed in an oblique orientation to obtain the entire length of the gallbladder. The neck, body, and fundus should be demonstrated (Fig. 4-6).
  - Scan completely through the gallbladder by angling the transducer or sliding it (i.e., medial to lateral), trying to maintain longitudinal orientation to the gallbladder.
  - Assess for the Murphy sign by applying transducer pressure to elicit possible associated discomfort.
  - Assess for intraluminal objects, like gallstones, polyps, or masses.
  - Assess for wall thickening and pericholecystic fluid.
- Transverse gallbladder (Fig. 4-7):
  - Images should be oriented 90° to the long axis of the gallbladder and thus the transducer may need to be placed in an oblique orientation to obtain these images.
  - Scan completely through the gallbladder by angling the transducer or sliding it (i.e., superior to inferior), trying to maintain transverse orientation to the gallbladder.
  - Transverse neck, body, and fundus should be evaluated. The neck should be located near the porta hepatis, and thus angling/sliding superiorly will demonstrate the neck, while angling/sliding inferiorly will demonstrate the fundus.
  - Assess for the Murphy sign by applying transducer pressure to elicit possible associated discomfort.
  - Assess for intraluminal objects, like gallstones, polyps, or masses.
  - Assess for wall thickening and pericholecystic fluid.
- Transverse or longitudinal gallbladder wall measurement (Figs. 4-8 and 4-9):
  - Some institutions prefer a transverse gallbladder wall measurement, while others prefer a longitudinal measurement.
  - Ensure that the transducer is perpendicular to the wall before obtaining a measurement. An oblique wall measurement may yield a false thickening.

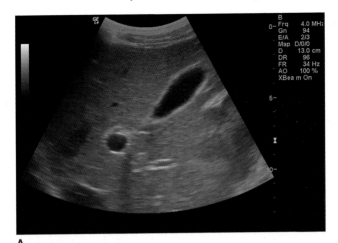

A

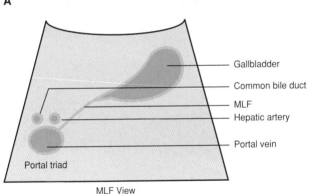

B

MLF View

**Figure 4-4. Main lobar fissure. The main lobar fissure can assist
in the identification of the gallbladder. A: It appears to connect the
gallbladder neck to the portal vein. B: Diagram demonstrating the
relationship of the main lobar fissure (MLF) and the gallbladder.**
(Reprinted with permission from Cosby KS, Kendall JL, eds. *Practical Guide
to Emergency Ultrasound.* 2nd ed. Philadelphia, PA: Wolters Kluwer Health/
Lippincott Williams & Wilkins; 2013.)

4. GB and Biliary

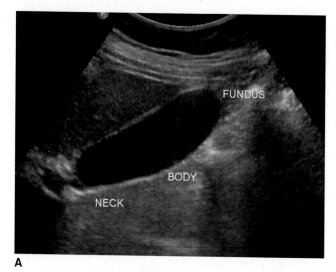

A

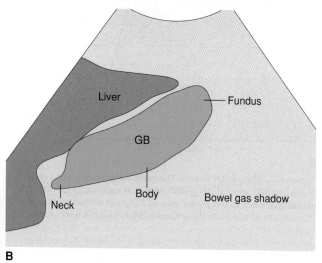

B

Figure 4-5. Longitudinal gallbladder. A,B: Longitudinal image of the gallbladder (GB) demonstrating the neck, body, and fundus.
(Part A is reprinted with permission from Kawamura D, Nolan T, eds. *Abdomen and Superficial Structures*. 4th ed. Philadelphia, PA: Wolters Kluwer; 2017.)

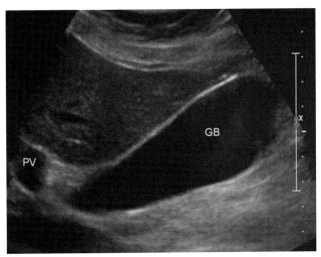

A

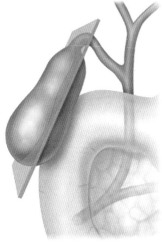

B

Figure 4-6. **Oblique orientation needed to obtain true longitudinal image of the gallbladder. A: Longitudinal image of the gallbladder. B: Drawing of the orientation often required to obtain a true longitudinal image of the gallbladder.** (Reprinted with permission from Kawamura D, Nolan T, eds. *Abdomen and Superficial Structures.* 4th ed. Philadelphia, PA: Wolters Kluwer; 2017.)

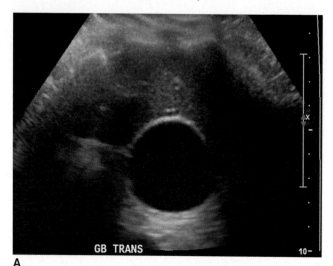

A

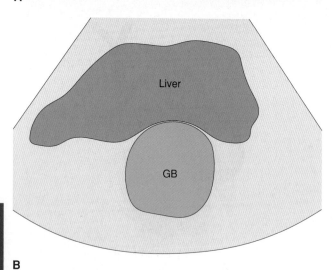

B

Figure 4-7. Transverse gallbladder. Transverse image of the gallbladder (GB) body. (Part A is reprinted with permission from Kawamura D, Nolan T, eds. *Abdomen and Superficial Structures*. 4th ed. Philadelphia, PA: Wolters Kluwer; 2017.)

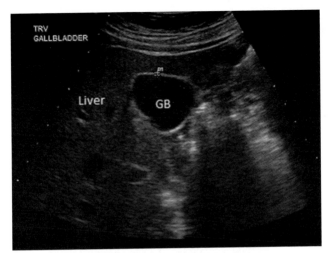

A

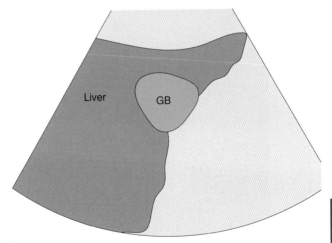

B

Figure 4-8. Transverse gallbladder wall measurement. A,B: Transverse image of the gallbladder (GB) and corresponding measurement of the gallbladder wall (between *calipers*).

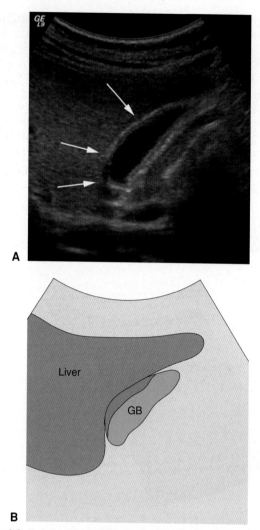

A

B

Figure 4-9. **Longitudinal gallbladder wall measurement. A,B: Longitudinal image of the gallbladder (GB; *arrows*) with a thickened wall.** (Part A is reprinted with permission from Kawamura D, Nolan T, eds. *Abdomen and Superficial Structures*. 4th ed. Philadelphia, PA: Wolters Kluwer; 2017.)

- Left lateral decubitus images:
  - Repeat longitudinal (see Fig. 4-5) and transverse (see Fig. 4-7) images of the gallbladder in the left lateral decubitus position.
  - Assess for intraluminal objects, like gallstones, polyps, or masses.
  - Assess for wall thickening and pericholecystic fluid.
- Additional images:
  - If the patient is capable, prone and upright images can be obtained to further evaluate the gallbladder.
- Bile ducts:
  - Long common duct:
    - The image should be oriented to the long axis of the porta hepatis to demonstrate the length of the common hepatic duct and common bile duct (**Fig. 4-10**).
    - Measurements of the ducts are obtained from the inner wall to the inner wall.
    - Typically, the common duct will be seen anterior to the hepatic artery, though this relationship may be reversed in some individuals (**Fig. 4-11**). Color Doppler will help in the identification of the common duct, because while the hepatic artery will demonstrate blood flow, the common duct will not.
    - Color Doppler can be used to demonstrate the intrahepatic ducts, though they are not typically seen (**Fig. 4-12**).
    - Lengthen the common bile duct as much as possible in order to assess it in its entirety, including the segment near the pancreatic head (**Fig. 4-13**).
    - Some interpreting physicians may require a measurement of the duct to be taken anterior to the hepatic artery (**Fig. 4-14**).

4. GB and Biliary

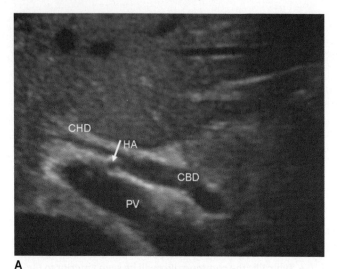

A

B

Figure 4-10. Longitudinal sonogram (A) and drawing (B) of the porta hepatis demonstrating the relationship of the common bile duct (CBD), hepatic artery (HA), and main portal vein (PV). (Reprinted with permission from Kawamura D, Nolan T, eds. *Abdomen and Superficial Structures*. 4th ed. Philadelphia, PA: Wolters Kluwer; 2017.)

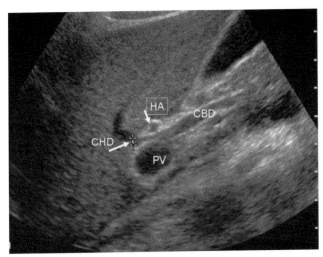

Figure 4-11. Reverse relationship of the common duct and hepatic artery. Occasionally, a replaced hepatic artery is seen. The artery is located anterior to the duct, rather than between the duct and portal vein. (Reprinted with permission from Kawamura D, Lunsford B, eds. *Abdomen and Superficial Structures.* 3rd ed. Philadelphia, PA: Wolters Kluwer Health/Lippincott Williams & Wilkins; 2012.)

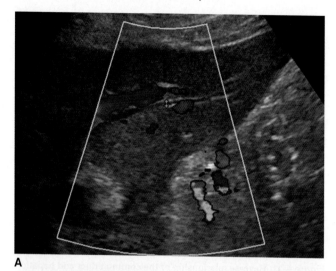

A

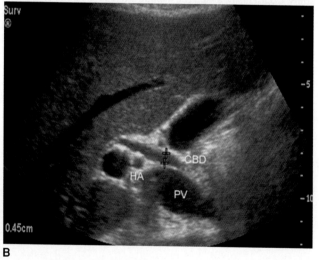

B

Figure 4-12. Normal measurements of the bile ducts. The ducts are measured inner wall to inner wall. A: Intrahepatic duct (between *calipers*). B: Common bile duct, <8 mm and (C) common hepatic duct, <6 mm at the porta hepatis.

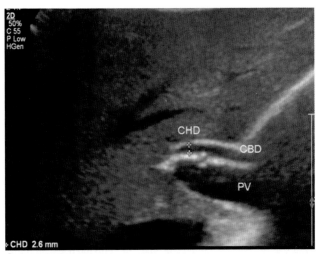

C

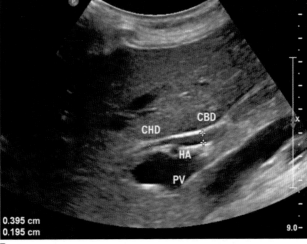

D

Figure 4-12 *(continued).* **D: Normal duct measurements at the porta hepatis. CBD, common bile duct measurement (between *calipers*); CHD, common hepatic duct; HA, hepatic artery; PV, portal vein.** (Reprinted with permission from Kawamura D, Nolan T, eds. *Abdomen and Superficial Structures.* 4th ed. Philadelphia, PA: Wolters Kluwer; 2017.)

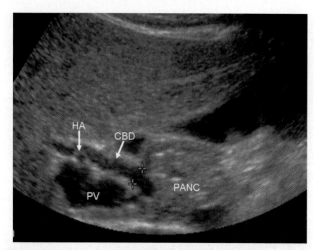

Figure 4-13. Distal common bile duct. The common bile duct (CBD) can be seen (between *calipers*) near the pancreatic head (PANC). **PV, portal vein; HA, hepatic artery.** (Reprinted with permission from Kawamura D, Lunsford B, eds. *Abdomen and Superficial Structures*. 3rd ed. Philadelphia, PA: Wolters Kluwer Health/Lippincott Williams & Wilkins; 2012.)

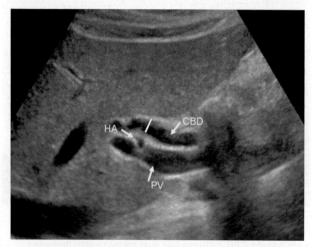

Figure 4-14. Measurement of the common duct anterior to the hepatic artery. (Reprinted with permission from Kawamura D, Lunsford B, eds. *Abdomen and Superficial Structures*. 3rd ed. Philadelphia, PA: Wolters Kluwer Health/Lippincott Williams & Wilkins; 2012.)

SCANNING TIPS

- Gallbladder:
  - Deep suspended inspiration will assist in displacing the gallbladder inferiorly.
  - Evaluate the gallbladder through the right-side rib windows when necessary. A smaller transducer face may be helpful.
  - If the gallbladder is not visualized:
    - Inquire about previous cholecystectomy
    - Inquire about fasting status
    - Possible WES (wall-echo-shadow) sign could be present, which occurs when the gallbladder is completely filled with gallstones and only the anterior wall of the gallbladder can be seen sonographically. A distinct shadow will be seen originating from the gallbladder fossa.
  - The gallbladder body and fundus can be mobile. In real time, actively scan the gallbladder while the patient changes positions.
  - Assess the gallbladder neck carefully for gallstones, because this is the most common location for gallstones to become lodged.
  - Gallstones will most likely be mobile and shadow, while polyps will not be mobile and should not shadow.
  - Gallbladder shape is variable.
    - The Phrygian cap is a fold in the fundus of the gallbladder (Fig. 4-15).
    - The junctional fold is a fold in the neck of the gallbladder (Fig. 4-16).
- Bile ducts:
  - Deep suspended inspiration will assist in displacing the liver inferiorly.
  - Left lateral decubitus or scanning through the right-side rib windows can aid in the assessment of the biliary tree.
  - Utilize color Doppler while analyzing the porta hepatis to differentiate the common duct from the hepatic artery.
  - If the biliary tract is dilated, try to follow the common bile duct over the head of the pancreas for signs of choledocholithiasis or possibly an obstructing pancreatic head mass.

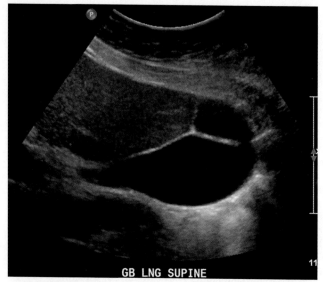

GB LNG SUPINE

Figure 4-15. The Phrygian cap. A Phrygian cap is a fold in the fundus of the gallbladder. (Reprinted with permission from Kawamura D, Nolan T, eds. *Abdomen and Superficial Structures*. 4th ed. Philadelphia, PA: Wolters Kluwer; 2017.)

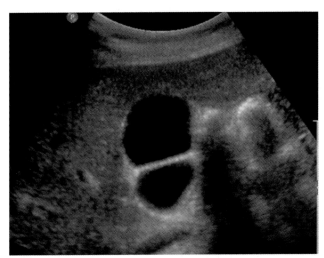

A

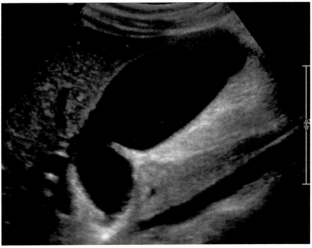

B

Figure 4-16. **Junctional fold. A junctional fold is a fold in the neck of the gallbladder. A: Transverse. B: Longitudinal.** (Reprinted with permission from Kawamura D, Lunsford B, eds. *Abdomen and Superficial Structures.* 3rd ed. Philadelphia, PA: Wolters Kluwer Health/Lippincott Williams & Wilkins; 2012.)

NORMAL MEASUREMENTS OF THE GALLBLADDER AND BILIARY TRACT

- Gallbladder[3]:
  - Size = 8–10 cm in length and 4–5 cm in diameter
  - Normal gallbladder wall thickness = <3 mm
- Biliary tract[2,3]:
  - Intrahepatic ducts diameter = <2 mm
  - Common hepatic duct diameter = <7–8 mm (depending on the patient's age and other factors)*
  - Common bile duct diameter = <7–8 mm (depending on patient's age and other factors)*
  - Bile duct wall thickness = <5 mm

ESSENTIAL GALLBLADDER AND BILIARY TRACT PATHOLOGY[2]

- Gallbladder pathology:
  - Cholelithiasis—gallstones
    - Clinical findings:
      ○ Asymptomatic
      ○ Biliary colic
      ○ Abdominal pain after high-fat meals
      ○ Epigastric pain
      ○ Nausea and vomiting
      ○ Shoulder or chest pain
    - Sonographic findings (Fig. 4-17):
      ○ Hyperechoic, mobile shadowing focus or foci
      ○ Evaluate for signs of cholecystitis (see this chapter heading Acute cholecystitis)
  - Gallbladder sludge:
    - Clinical findings:
      ○ Asymptomatic
      ○ Biliary stasis (extended amount of time fasting, TPN)
    - Sonographic findings (Fig. 4-18):
      ○ Layering low-level, nonshadowing, dependent echoes within the gallbladder

---

*Bile duct diameter can be larger after cholecystectomy and the diameter may increase with age. Both imaging and clinical assessment must be correlated when ductal dilatation is suspected.

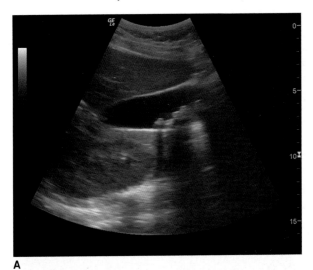

A

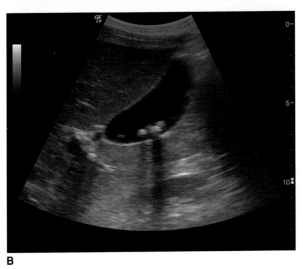

B

Figure 4-17. **Mobility of gallstones. A: Multiple gallstones are noted in the fundus of the gallbladder. B: The gallstones have moved with a change in patient positioning.** (Reprinted with permission from Cosby KS, Kendall JL, eds. *Practical Guide to Emergency Ultrasound.* 2nd ed. Philadelphia, PA: Wolters Kluwer Health/Lippincott Williams & Wilkins; 2013.)

4. GB and Biliary

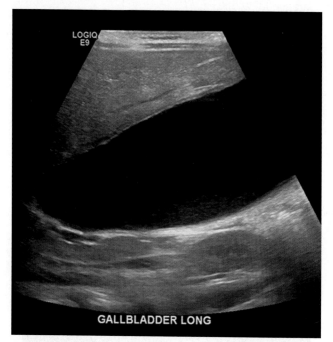

Figure 4-18. Gallbladder sludge. (Image courtesy of Philips Healthcare, Bothell, WA.)

- Gallbladder polyps:
  - Clinical findings:
    - Asymptomatic
  - Sonographic findings **(Fig. 4-19)**:
    - Hyperechoic, nonshadowing, and nonmobile focus or foci attached to the gallbladder wall that project within the lumen
    - Polyps measuring over 1 cm could be suggestive of gallbladder carcinoma
- Adenomyomatosis—accumulation of cholesterol crystals within the gallbladder wall:
  - Clinical findings:
    - Asymptomatic

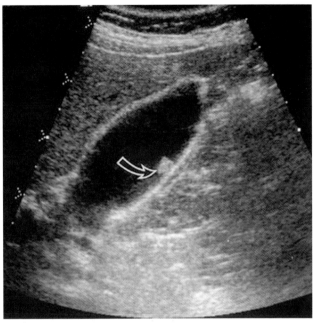

Figure 4-19. Gallbladder polyp. A polyp (*arrow*) is noted within this gallbladder. (Reprinted with permission from Yamada T, Alpers DH, Laine L, Kaplowitz N, Owyang C, Powell DW, eds. *Textbook of Gastroenterology.* 4th ed. Philadelphia, PA: Lippincott Williams & Wilkins; 2003.)

- Sonographic findings (**Fig. 4-20**):
  - Focal gallbladder wall thickening with evidence of comet-tail artifact emanating from the wall
- Acute cholecystitis—inflammation of the gallbladder:
  - Clinical findings:
    - Right upper quadrant, epigastric, or possibly shoulder or chest pain
    - Elevation in WBC, ALP, ALT, GGT, and possibly bilirubin with obstruction
    - Fever
    - Nausea and vomiting

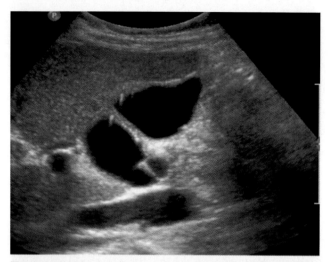

Figure 4-20. Adenomyomatosis. Comet tail artifact is noted emanating from the wall of the anterior gallbladder, which indicates the presence of adenomyomatosis. (Reprinted with permission from Kawamura D, Lunsford B, eds. *Abdomen and Superficial Structures*. 3rd ed. Philadelphia, PA: Wolters Kluwer Health/Lippincott Williams & Wilkins; 2012.)

- Sonographic findings (Fig. 4-21):
  - Gallstones*
  - Positive Murphy sign
  - Gallbladder wall thickening
  - Gallbladder enlargement (hydrops)
  - Pericholecystic fluid
  - Sludge
- Biliary tract pathology:
  - Choledocholithiasis—gallstone within the biliary duct(s):
    - Clinical findings:
      - Right upper quadrant pain
      - Jaundice
      - Elevated ALP, ALT, GGT, and bilirubin with obstruction
    - Sonographic findings (Fig. 4-22):
      - Hyperechoic, shadowing focus or foci within the bile duct(s)

---

*Patients can have acalculous cholecystitis as well, in which all clinical and sonographic signs are present though no gallstones are seen.

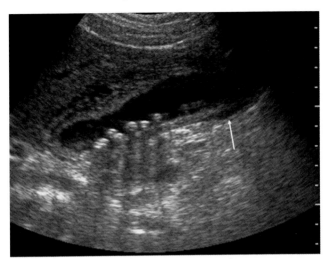

A

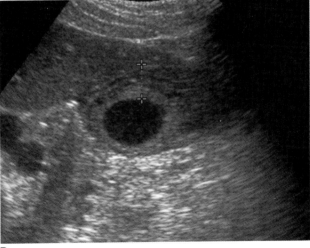

B

Figure 4-21. Acute cholecystitis. A: Longitudinal image in a patient with a positive Murphy sign. Note the gallstones, sludge, thickened, edematous wall, and pericholecystic fluid (*arrow*). B: Transverse image of another patient with acute cholecystitis and thickened wall (*calipers*). *(continued)*

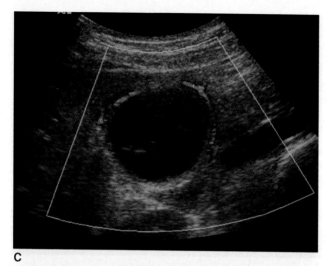

C

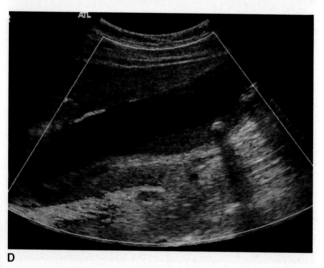

D

Figure 4-21 *(continued).* **C: Hydropic gallbladder and increased color Doppler flow in a patient with positive Murphy sign, sludge, and acute cholecystitis. D: Longitudinal image of acute cholecystitis, stone, sludge, and increased Doppler flow.** (Reprinted with permission from Kawamura D, Nolan T, eds. *Abdomen and Superficial Structures.* 4th ed. Philadelphia, PA: Wolters Kluwer; 2017.)

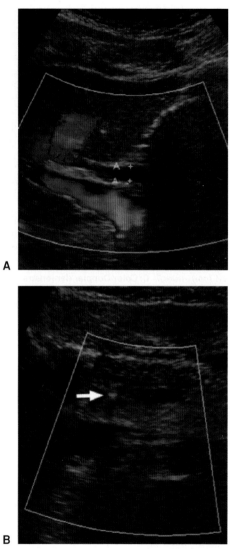

A

B

Figure 4-22. Choledocholithiasis. A: Longitudinal sonogram reveals a dilated common bile duct (CBD) (between *calipers*) measuring 7 mm in diameter in a young patient. B: A 4-mm echogenic, shadowing focus (*arrow*) is seen at the level of the pancreatic head. *(continued)*

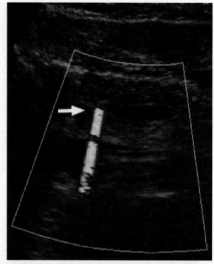

C

**Figure 4-22 *(continued).* C: Color Doppler demonstrates the
twinkle sign posterior to the stone.** (Reprinted with permission from
Lee E, ed. *Pediatric Radiology: Practical Imaging Evaluation of Infants and
Children.* Philadelphia, PA: Wolters Kluwer; 2017.)

- Possible dilatation of the biliary tree and enlargement
  of the gallbladder
- Color Doppler applied over the area of the stone will
  reveal twinkle artifact (see Fig. 4-22C)
- Cholangitis—inflammation of the bile ducts:
  - Clinical findings:
    - Fever
    - Right upper quadrant pain
    - Jaundice
    - Elevated WBC, ALP, ALT, GGT, and bilirubin with
      obstruction
  - Sonographic findings (Fig. 4-23):
    - Biliary dilatation
    - Sludge
    - Thickening of the bile duct walls
    - Possible choledocholithiasis

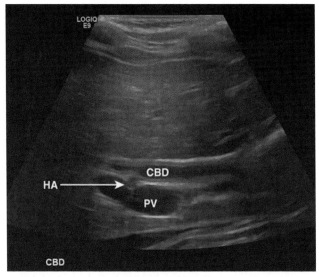

Figure 4-23. Cholangitis. Note the thickened wall of the common bile duct (CBD). HA, hepatic artery; PV, portal vein. (Reprinted with permission from Kawamura D, Lunsford B, eds. *Abdomen and Superficial Structures.* 3rd ed. Philadelphia, PA: Wolters Kluwer Health/Lippincott Williams & Wilkins; 2012.)

WHERE ELSE TO LOOK

- Analyze the liver first for signs of intrahepatic biliary dilatation.
- Keep in mind, that biliary dilatation typically occurs proximal to the level of obstruction, so if dilatation is present, ensure that the entire length of the common bile duct is assessed.
- Evaluate the pancreatic head carefully for signs of a mass, especially when there is evidence of biliary dilatation or gallbladder enlargement.

IMAGE CORRELATION

- Gallstones on CT (**Fig. 4-24**)
- Acute cholecystitis on CT (**Fig. 4-25**)

4. GB and Biliary

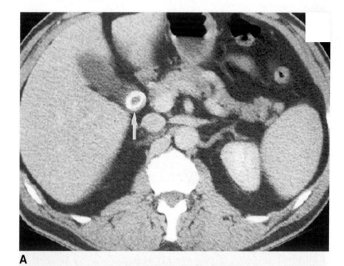

A

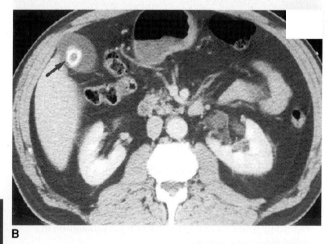

B

Figure 4-24. **Incidental gallstones on CT. A:** Enhanced CT image shows a rim-calcified, oval gallstone (*arrow*) lodged in the gallbladder neck. **B:** Image through the gallbladder fundus shows a large, faceted stone (*arrow*) in the gallbladder fundus in the same patient.

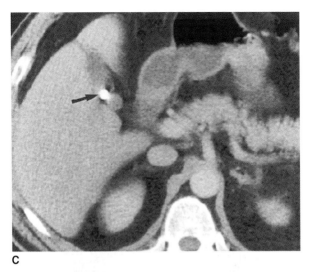

C

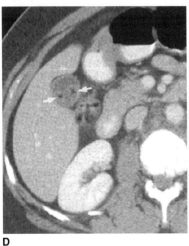

D

Figure 4-24 *(continued)*. C: Image through the gallbladder neck in a different patient shows a 9-mm, uniformly calcified stone (*arrow*) in the gallbladder neck. D: Image through the gallbladder fundus in a third patient shows gas-filled gallstones (*arrows*). (Reprinted with permission from Pope TL Jr, Harris JH Jr, eds. *Harris & Harris' The Radiology of Emergency Medicine.* 5th ed. Philadelphia, PA: Wolters Kluwer Health/ Lippincott Williams & Wilkins; 2012.)

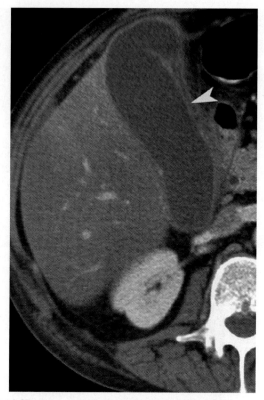

Figure 4-25. Cholecystitis on CT. Contrast-enhanced CT demonstrating gallbladder wall thickening and pericholecystic fluid (*arrowhead*) from acute cholecystitis. (Reprinted with permission from Singh A. *Gastrointestinal Imaging: The Essentials*. Philadelphia, PA: Wolters Kluwer; 2016.)

REFERENCES

1. AIUM practice parameters for the performance of an ultrasound of the abdomen and/or retroperitoneum. http://www.aium.org/resources/guidelines/abdominal.pdf. Accessed June 27, 2018.
2. Penny SM, ed. *Examination Review for Ultrasound: Abdomen & Obstetrics and Gynecology.* 2nd ed. Philadelphia, PA: Wolters Kluwer; 2018:1–78.
3. Kawamura DM, Nolan TD, eds. *Diagnostic Medical Sonography: Abdomen and Superficial Structures.* 4th ed. Philadelphia, PA: Wolters Kluwer; 2018: 171–212.
4. Hopkins TB. *Lab Notes: Guide to Lab and Diagnostic Tests.* 2nd ed. Philadelphia, PA: F. A. Davis Company; 2009.

CHAPTER 5

Urinary Tract

INTRODUCTION

Sonography of the urinary tract is a commonly requested examination. In fact, there are many disorders of the urinary tract in which sonography can provide a vital initial imaging screening. And thus, a thorough routine protocol must be established in order to identify pathology of the urinary tract. This chapter will provide essential anatomy and physiology, protocol, anomalies, and pathology of the adult urinary tract. Relevant clinical findings, including laboratory findings, are also provided.

AIUM RECOMMENDATIONS FOR SONOGRAPHY OF THE URINARY TRACT[1]

- Assess the urinary tract in the following manner:
  - Kidneys (including vascular assessment and adrenal glands):
    - The sonographic evaluation of the kidneys should include long-axis and transverse views.
    - A measurement of the maximum length of the kidneys should be obtained.
    - Decubitus, prone, or upright positioning may be helpful to better evaluate the kidneys.
    - The echogenicity of the right kidney should be compared to the echogenicity of the liver, while the echogenicity of the left kidney should be compared to that of the spleen.
    - Renal cortical thickness should be evaluated.
    - The renal cortices, sinuses, renal pelves, and perirenal region should be evaluated for signs of abnormalities, including dilatation of the collecting system, calculi, and masses.
    - Color Doppler may be used to detect calculi via the twinkle artifact.

- Vascular assessment of the kidneys should include:
  - The renal artery and renal vein should be evaluated for patency.
  - For suspected renal artery stenosis, angle-adjusted measurements of the peak systolic velocity of the proximal, central, and distal portions of the extrarenal main renal artery should be used when possible.
  - The peak systolic velocity of the adjacent abdominal aorta should be documented for calculating the ratio of the renal to aortic peak systolic velocity.
  - Spectral Doppler evaluation of the intrarenal arteries may be helpful for providing an indirect sign of proximal stenosis in the main renal artery.
- Urinary Bladder:
  - Transverse and longitudinal images of the distended urinary bladder should be provided.
  - An evaluation of intraluminal and wall abnormalities should be provided.
  - The distal ureter should be assessed for abnormalities, including obtaining ureteral jets with color Doppler imaging when a urinary tract obstruction is suspected.
  - In women, transvaginal imaging may be utilized to evaluate for distal ureteral stones.
  - Transverse and longitudinal images of the postvoid residual can provide a quantitative analysis.
  - The male prostate gland may be measured and incidental gynecologic findings should be noted.
- Adrenal glands:
  - The adrenal gland area should be evaluated in the adult, although normal adrenal glands are less commonly seen in older children and adults.
  - Any masses should be documented.
  - Longitudinal and transverse images of the adrenal glands in newborns and young infants may be obtained, especially when clinically indicated.

ESSENTIAL ANATOMY AND PHYSIOLOGY OF THE URINARY TRACT

- The urinary tract consists of the kidneys, ureters, bladder, and urethra.

- Kidney anatomy and physiology:
  - The paired kidneys are bean-shaped, retroperitoneal organs located in the posterior aspect of the right and left upper quadrants (Figs. 5-1 and 5-2).
  - Each kidney consists of two parts, which are the renal parenchyma and the renal sinus.
    - The renal parenchyma includes the renal medulla and the renal cortex, and it includes the renal pyramids.
    - The renal sinus includes the renal collecting system, including the calices and the renal pelvis.
  - The kidney can be divided into an upper or superior pole, midportion, which includes the renal hilum, and a lower or inferior pole.
  - The kidneys perform many vital functions, including detoxification and filtration of the blood, blood pressure regulation, and maintaining normal pH, iron, and salt levels in the blood.
  - There are several renal variants that may alter the appearance of the kidney (Table 5-1).
- Ureteral anatomy:
  - The bilateral ureters are small tubes that connect the kidney to the bladder.
  - The proximal ureter unites with the renal pelvis at the ureteropelvic junction (UPJ).
  - The distal ureter unites with the bladder at the ureterovesicular junction (UVJ).
  - The ureters provide a means whereby urine can travel from the kidneys to the urinary bladder.
- Bladder and urethral anatomy:
  - The urinary bladder, located in the anterior pelvis, is a temporary storage organ for urine.

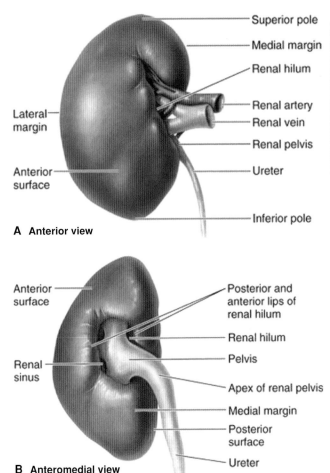

Superior pole

Medial margin

Renal hilum

Renal artery

Renal vein

Renal pelvis

Ureter

Inferior pole

Lateral margin

Anterior surface

A Anterior view

Anterior surface

Posterior and anterior lips of renal hilum

Renal hilum

Pelvis

Apex of renal pelvis

Medial margin

Posterior surface

Ureter

Renal sinus

B Anteromedial view

Figure 5-1. **External and internal appearance of kidneys. A: The right kidney. B: Renal sinus, as seen through the renal hilum.** *(continued)*

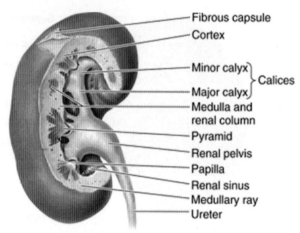

C Anterior view exposing calices

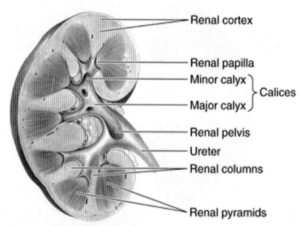

D Anterior view, coronal section

Figure 5-1 *(continued)*. **C:** The anterior lip of the renal hilum has been cut away to expose the renal pelvis and calices within the renal sinus. **D:** This coronal section of the kidney shows the organ's internal structure. The renal pyramids contain the collecting tubules and form the medulla of the kidney. The renal cortex contains the **renal corpuscles.** (Reprinted with permission from Moore KL, Dalley AF, Agur AM, eds. *Clinically Oriented Anatomy.* 7th ed. Philadelphia, PA: Wolters Kluwer Health/Lippincott Williams & Wilkins; 2013.)

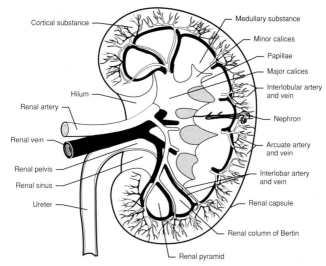

Figure 5-2. Kidney anatomy including vascularity. (Reprinted with permission from Penny SM, ed. *Examination Review for Ultrasound*. Philadelphia, PA: Wolters Kluwer Health/Lippincott Williams & Wilkins; 2010.)

Table 5-1 RENAL VARIANTS AND DESCRIPTION

MOST COMMON RENAL VARIANTS	DESCRIPTION
Duplex collecting system (Fig. 5-3)	Two separate renal sinuses with separate collecting systems
Junctional line (or junctional parenchymal defect) (Fig. 5-4)	An echogenic line or triangular structure most likely in the upper pole of the kidney that results from the fusion of two parenchymal renal embryonic renunculi
Dromedary hump (Fig. 5-5)	Bulge on the lateral border of the kidney, often on the left kidney
Ectopic kidney (pelvic kidney)	A kidney in the wrong locations, most often in the pelvis
Extrarenal pelvis (Fig. 5-6)	The renal pelvis is located outside of the renal hilum
Horseshoe kidneys (Fig. 5-7)	Two kidneys that cross the midline and attach at the lower poles by a bridge of tissue called an isthmus

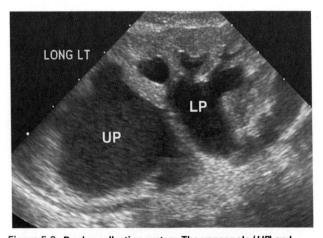

Figure 5-3. Duplex collecting system. The upper pole (*UP*) and lower pole (*LP*) contain separate dilated renal collecting systems.
(Reprinted with permission from Siegel MJ, Coley B, eds. *Core Curriculum: Pediatric Imaging.* Philadelphia, PA: Lippincott Williams & Wilkins; 2005.)

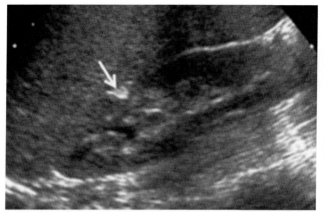

A

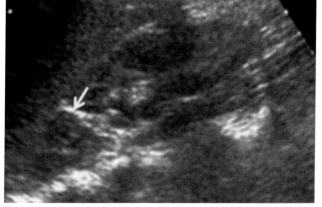

B

Figure 5-4. Junctional line. A, B: A junctional parenchymal defect or line (*arrows*) is noted in these kidneys. (Reprinted with permission from Siegel MJ, ed. *Pediatric Sonography*. 4th ed. Philadelphia, PA: Wolters Kluwer Health/Lippincott Williams & Wilkins; 2010.)

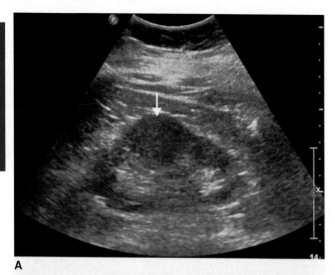

A

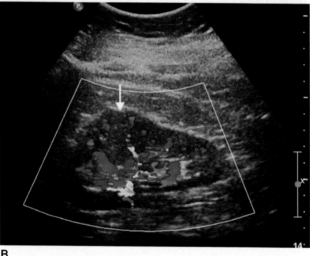

B

Figure 5-5. **Dromedary hump. A, B: A dromedary hump (*arrow*) is noted in these images as extrarenal tissue in the midportion of the kidney.** (Reprinted with permission from Sanders RC, ed. *Clinical Sonography: A Practical Guide.* 5th ed. Philadelphia, PA: Wolters Kluwer; 2015.)

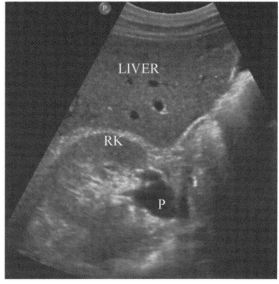

Figure 5-6. Extrarenal pelvis. The renal pelvis (*P*) is located outside of the renal hilum in this right kidney (*RK*). (Reprinted with permission from Kawamura D, Nolan T, eds. *Abdomen and Superficial Structures*. 4th ed. Philadelphia, PA: Wolters Kluwer; 2017.)

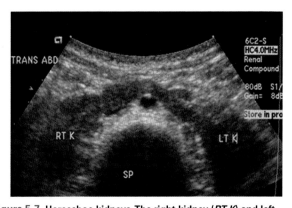

Figure 5-7. Horseshoe kidneys. The right kidney (*RT K*) and left kidney (*LT K*) are attached by a thin band of tissue, the isthmus, which is noted in this image anterior to the spine (*SP*). (Reprinted with permission from MacDonald MG, Seshia MM, eds. *Avery's Neonatology*. 7th ed. Philadelphia, PA: Wolters Kluwer; 2015.)

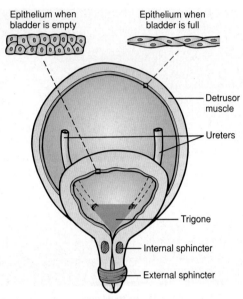

Figure 5-8. Basic urinary bladder anatomy. (Reprinted with permission from Porth C, ed. *Essentials of Pathophysiology.* 4th ed. Philadelphia, PA: Wolters Kluwer; 2014.)

- The bladder includes an area referred to as the trigone, which is where the two UVJs and the opening for the urethra are located (**Fig. 5-8**).
- The urethra is a tube that extends from the trigone of the bladder to the outside of the body.
- Voiding or urination is the process of allowing urine to exit the bladder through the urethra.

PATIENT PREPARATION FOR SONOGRAPHY OF THE URINARY TRACT

- There is typically no patient preparation for a sonogram of the urinary tract. However, some institutions may require that the patient be well hydrated.
- A distended urinary bladder is warranted to best evaluate for intraluminal abnormalities and wall thickening.

SUGGESTED EQUIPMENT[1]

- 3.5–5-MHz transducer:
  - Higher frequencies can be used for thin patients, and a small-footprint transducer may be required to visualize through narrow intercostal spaces.
- General abdominal or renal setting (most machines)
- Positional sponges for decubitus images

CLINICAL INVESTIGATION FOR SONOGRAPHY OF THE URINARY TRACT[2]

- Laboratory values are listed in Table 5-2:
  - Evaluate prior imaging reports and images including CT, MRI, radiography, and any other appropriate tests.
- Critical clinical history questions related to the urinary tract:
  - History of urinary tract infection(s)? *Recurring urinary tract infections can damage the kidneys. Also, an analysis for signs of kidney stones, pyelonephritis, thickening of the urinary bladder wall, and debris in the renal collecting system or urinary bladder should take place.*
  - History of nephrectomy or other urinary tract surgery (e.g., bladder surgery)? *Not only will the kidney be absent, but the motive for the previous nephrectomy may be relevant. For example, a history of renal cell carcinoma is valuable information to obtain because a detailed analysis of the remaining kidney for signs of carcinoma should commence.*
  - History of kidney stones? *A careful analysis for evidence of stones should be conducted, especially if clinical symptoms are suggestive.*
  - History of diabetes mellitus or high blood pressure? *Diabetes and high blood pressure can damage the function of the kidneys. The structure, and thus the sonographic appearance of the kidneys may also be altered with uncontrolled diabetes and/or high blood pressure.*
  - History of blood in the urine (gross or microscopic hematuria)? *Hematuria can be a sign of renal stones, infection, or even malignancy.*
  - History of renal anomalies? *Some individuals may be aware that they have duplicated collecting systems, unilateral renal agenesis, or horseshoe kidneys.*

Table 5-2	LAB AND URINALYSIS FINDINGS AND POSSIBLE ASSOCIATED URINARY TRACT PATHOLOGY

LAB FINDING	POTENTIAL PATHOLOGY
↑ WBC (leukocytosis)	Urinary tract infection or inflammation
↓ WBC (leukopenia)	Chemotherapy, radiation therapy, toxic reaction
↓ Hematocrit	Acute hemorrhage
↑ Blood urea nitrogen (BUN)	Renal failure, renal parenchymal disease, urinary tract obstruction, dehydration, diabetes mellitus, hemorrhage
↓ Blood urea nitrogen (BUN)	Liver disease, malnutrition, overhydration, smoking, pregnancy
↑ Creatinine	Renal failure, chronic nephritis, urinary tract obstruction, diabetes mellitus, compromised renal blood flow
↓ Glomerular filtration rate (GFR)	Renal insufficiency or chronic renal disease
↑ Lactate dehydrogenase (LDH)	Renal infarction or chronic renal disease
↑ Bacteria (bacteriuria)	Acute pyelonephritis or urinary tract infection
Pyuria	Urinary tract infection
Hematuria	Acute or chronic pyelonephritis, calculi, renal cell carcinoma, renal infarction, or trauma
↑ Protein (proteinuria)	Urinary tract infection, glomerulo-nephritis, urinary tract masses, nephrotic syndrome, pyelonephritis, or calculi
↑ Specific gravity	Dehydration
↓ Specific gravity	Renal failure and pyelonephritis

NORMAL SONOGRAPHIC DESCRIPTION OF THE URINARY TRACT

• The normal kidneys appear as bean-shaped organs. The cortex typically appears to consist of medium- to low-level echoes, while the sinus has more of an echogenic appearance. The kidney cortices should either be isoechoic or more hypoechoic than the normal liver or spleen.

- The ureters are not typically seen sonographically. If the ureters are noted, an investigation for urinary obstruction should be conducted.
- In the distended state, the urinary bladder appears as an anechoic structure outlined by a thin hyperechoic wall. In transverse, the distended urinary bladder may appear as a square-shaped, anechoic structure within the pelvis.
- The UVJs may be demonstrated best in transverse as small bilateral bulges in the inferoposterior aspect of the urinary bladder wall.

SUGGESTED PROTOCOL FOR SONOGRAPHY OF THE URINARY TRACT[1]

- Survey the kidney:
  - Start on the right side of the patient and complete the entire kidney protocol before moving to the left kidney or bladder.
  - Ask the patient to extend his or her left arms up above his or her head in order to expand the intercostal spaces.
    - Suspended or deep inspiration may be helpful to evaluate the kidneys.
  - With the patient in the supine position, obtain a brief survey of the kidney by scanning superiorly and inferiorly (transverse) or medial to lateral (longitudinal).
  - Evaluate the renal cortices, sinuses, renal pelves, and perirenal region for signs of abnormalities, including dilatation of the collecting system, calculi, and masses.
  - Perform a cine clip in longitudinal and transverse **(Video 5-1 and Video 5-2).**
- Longitudinal (right or left) kidney (repeat on contralateral side):
  - Lengthen the kidney in the longitudinal plane, which may require the transducer to be slightly obliqued.
  - Note the echogenicity of the kidney compared to the liver or spleen.
  - Ensure that the cortex is clearly visualized around the sinus.

- Measure the length of the kidney (Fig. 5-9).
  - An anteroposterior dimension of the kidney may be obtained as well.
- If requested, apply color Doppler to the kidney to demonstrate vascular sufficiency. Also, color Doppler can assist in the identification of small renal calculi by demonstrating the twinkle sign or artifact.
- Longitudinal (right or left) kidney medial (repeat on contralateral side):
  - Obtain an image of the medial aspect of the kidney, noting the area of the renal pelvis.
  - Assess the area of the adrenal glands, which in adults are most likely located medial to the upper pole of each kidney.
- Longitudinal (right or left) kidney lateral (repeat on contralateral side):
  - Obtain an image of the lateral aspect of the kidney.
- Transverse (right or left) kidney upper pole (repeat on contralateral side):
  - Rotate the transducer 90° to the image of the kidney that was obtained in longitudinal and begin by evaluating the upper or superior pole of the kidney (Fig. 5-10).
  - Scan completely through the kidney superiorly in transverse.
- Transverse (right or left) kidney mid (repeat on contralateral side):
  - The renal hilum will appear as a section where the kidney tissue is disrupted medially by the renal vasculature. Therefore, the midportion of the kidney often appears as a "C."
  - Color Doppler may be applied to the kidney at the renal hilum level in order to demonstrate the renal vasculature and to differentiate these blood vessels from a prominent or dilated renal pelvis (Fig. 5-11).
  - The thickness of the kidney should be measured, if requested (Fig. 5-12).
- Transverse (right or left) kidney lower pole (repeat on contralateral side):
  - Image the lower or inferior pole of the kidney (Fig. 5-13).
  - Scan completely through the kidney inferiorly in transverse.

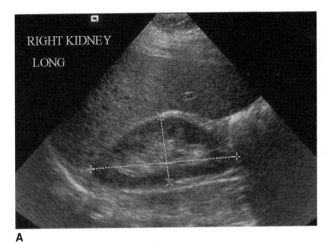

A

B

Figure 5-9. Longitudinal kidney with length measurement (A and drawing B). (Part A reprinted with permission from Kawamura D, Nolan T, eds. *Abdomen and Superficial Structures.* 4th ed. Philadelphia, PA: Wolters Kluwer; 2017.)

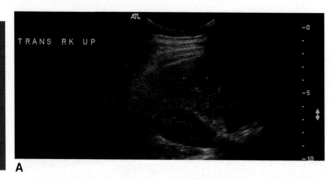

A

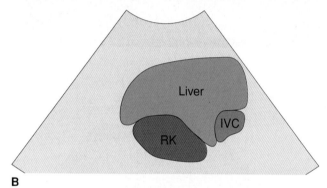

B

Figure 5-10. Transverse upper pole kidney image. In this image, the upper pole of the right kidney (*RK*) can be noted adjacent to the inferior vena cava (*IVC*) and posterior to the right lobe of the liver (A and drawing B).

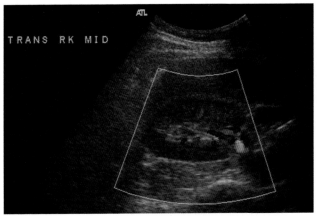

A

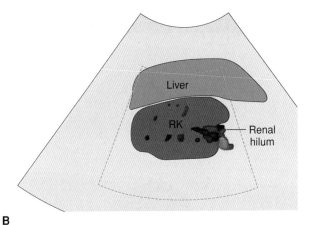

B

Figure 5-11. Transverse mid kidney image with color Doppler (A and drawing B).

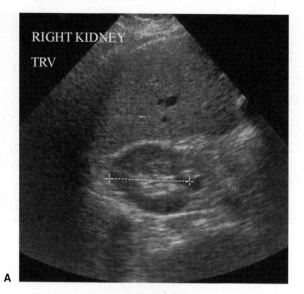

A

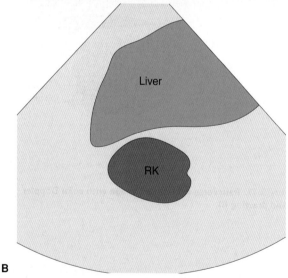

B

Figure 5-12. Transverse mid kidney image with measurement (A and drawing B). (Part A reprinted with permission from Kawamura D, Nolan T, eds. *Abdomen and Superficial Structures.* 4th ed. Philadelphia, PA: Wolters Kluwer; 2017.)

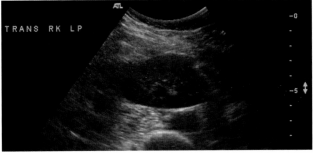

A

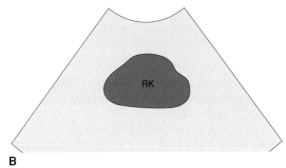

B

Figure 5-13. **Transverse lower pole kidney image. In this image, the upper pole of the right kidney (*RK*) can be noted adjacent to the inferior vena cava (*IVC*) and posterior to the right lobe of the liver (A and drawing B).**

- Survey the urinary bladder:
  - With the patient in the supine position, obtain a brief survey of the kidney by scanning superiorly and inferiorly (transverse) or anterior to posterior (longitudinal).
  - Obtain a video clip of the urinary bladder, if requested.
- Longitudinal urinary bladder:
  - Image the bladder in the longitudinal plane (Fig. 5-14).
  - Scanning medial to lateral completely through the bladder, evaluate the lumen of the urinary bladder and the urinary bladder wall.
- Transverse urinary bladder:
  - Image the bladder in the transverse plane (Fig. 5-14).

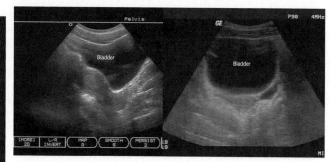

Figure 5-14. Longitudinal and transverse images of the urinary bladder. The longitudinal image is on the left and the transverse image is on the right. (Reprinted with permission from Cosby KS, Kendall JL, eds. *Practical Guide to Emergency Ultrasound.* 2nd ed. Philadelphia, PA: Wolters Kluwer Health/Lippincott Williams & Wilkins; 2013.)

- Scanning superior to inferior completely through the bladder, evaluate the lumen of the urinary bladder and the urinary bladder wall.
- Transverse bladder (with color Doppler):
  - The trigone of the bladder is located posteroinferior in the bladder.
  - Apply color Doppler to the trigone region of the urinary bladder.
  - Demonstrate ureteral patency by providing ureteral jet images of both UVJs. Color Doppler should be seen emanating from each UVJ **(Fig. 5-15).**
- Additional images:
  - Some institutions may require measurements of the renal cortex for signs of cortical thinning. In the longitudinal plane, measure from the outer border of the renal cortex to the outer border of the renal sinus.
  - Prevoid and postvoid residual bladder volumes can be obtained. To acquire these images, obtain a longitudinal and transverse image and measure in three dimensions.
  - Some institutions may request an analysis of the abdominal aorta for signs of abdominal aortic aneurysms and other vascular abnormalities.
  - After identifying hydronephrosis, postvoid images of the bladder and kidneys can provide further information.

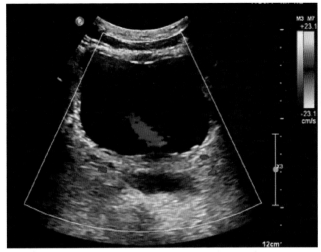

Figure 5-15. Transverse image of the urinary bladder with color Doppler demonstrating ureteral jets. In this image, only the left ureteral jet can be seen. (Reprinted with permission from Dunnick NR, Newhouse JH, Cohan RH, Maturen KE, eds. *Genitourinary Radiology*. 6th ed. Philadelphia, PA: Wolters Kluwer; 2017.)

SCANNING TIPS

- Don't be too quick to place the patient in decubitus positions to examine the kidneys, because in some individuals, the kidneys may be evaluated more readily in the supine position.
- Deep inspiration may help to visualize the kidneys in some patients, while in others, simply suspended breathing may help.
- A small-footprint transducer may be better to demonstrate the kidneys in thin patients with narrow intercostal spaces.
- Scanning posteriorly through the back muscles may be helpful in pediatric patients.
- Be careful to not misidentify an enlarged prostate as a bladder mass.
- Transvaginal imaging may be utilized to evaluate for distal ureteral stones in women.

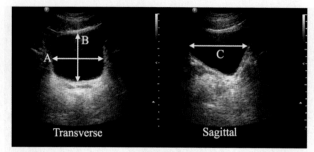

Figure 5-16. Obtaining a bladder volume. Scanning the bladder in the transverse and sagittal or longitudinal planes, identifying the largest diameters, and applying the formula Bladder volume = $(A \times B \times C \times 0.52)$ allows estimation of bladder volume in mL. A = bladder width (cm), B = bladder height (cm), C = bladder length (cm). (Reprinted with permission from Barash PG, Cahalan MK, Cullen BF, et al., eds. *Clinical Anesthesia.* 8th ed. Philadelphia, PA: Wolters Kluwer; 2017.)

NORMAL MEASUREMENTS OF THE URINARY TRACT[*][2-5]

- Renal length (adults):
  - 8–13 cm in length
  - 2–3 cm in anteroposterior dimension
  - 4–5 cm in width
- Renal volume:
  - Length × Width × Height × 0.523 = mL
- Renal cortex (adults):
  - 1 cm or more
- Bladder volume: (Fig. 5-16)
  - Length × Width × Height × 0.52 = mL
  - Bladder capacity is between 150–600 mL
- Bladder wall thickness:
  - 3 mm or less when distended
  - 5 mm or less when empty

ESSENTIAL URINARY TRACT PATHOLOGY[2]

- Hydronephrosis—dilation of the renal collecting system (Fig. 5-17):

---

*Renal size varies with age, gender, and other factors. Therefore, be careful to assess the entire clinical account when evaluating the size of the kidneys. For example, an evaluation of the laboratory values and other clinical history should be performed routinely, if possible, before claiming that the kidneys are either too large or too small.

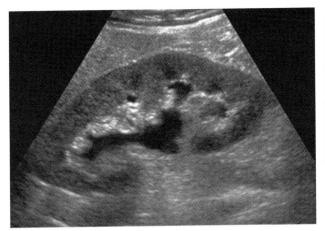

A

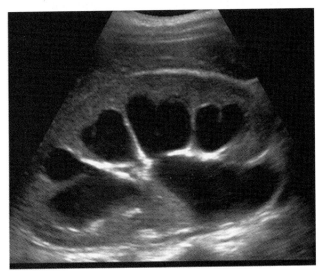

B

Figure 5-17. Hydronephrosis. Two longitudinal images of hydronephrotic kidneys. A. Mild hydronephrosis. B. Moderate hydronephrosis. (Reprinted with permission from Kawamura D, Nolan T, eds. *Abdomen and Superficial Structures.* 4th ed. Philadelphia, PA: Wolters Kluwer; 2017.)

- Common causes of hydronephrosis include the following:
  - Urolithiasis
  - UPJ or UVJ obstruction
  - Ureterocele: ballooning of the ureter into the bladder
  - Benign prostatic hypertrophy
  - Pregnancy
  - Pelvic masses: ovarian tumor or uterine fibroids
- Clinical findings:
  - May be asymptomatic
  - Could have signs or symptoms based on the cause of obstruction such as hematuria or pain when associated with a urolithiasis
- Sonographic findings:
  - Distention of the renal collecting system with anechoic fluid
  - Possible dilation of the ureter and enlargement of the bladder depending upon the level of obstruction
- Urolithiasis **(Fig. 5-18)**:
  - Clinical findings:
    - Hematuria
    - Renal colic: pain in the area of the stone
    - Oliguria
    - Urinary tract infection
  - Sonographic findings:
    - Echogenic focus that produces acoustic shadowing
    - Evidence of the "twinkle sign" or "twinkle artifact": increased Doppler artifact posterior to the stone
    - Hydronephrosis and/or dilation of the ureter proximal to the stone may be present
- Renal cysts—anechoic mass(es) within or on the kidney that produce posterior enhancement **(Fig. 5-19)**:
  - Autosomal dominant polycystic kidney disease:
    - Clinical findings:
      - Asymptomatic until third or fourth decade of life
      - Decreased renal function
      - Urinary tract infections
      - Renal stones
      - Flank pain
      - Hematuria
      - Palpable abdominal mass (representing enlarged kidney)

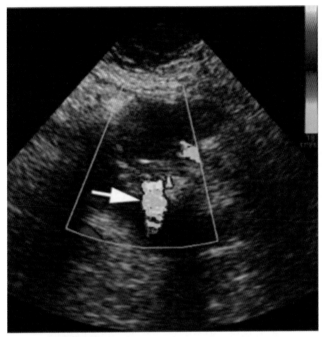

Figure 5-18. Urolithiasis with twinkle sign. Kidney stone (*arrows*) demonstrating the twinkle sign, which is described as increased color Doppler signal posterior to a stone. (Reprinted with permission from Siegel MJ, ed. *Pediatric Sonography.* 4th ed. Philadelphia, PA: Wolters Kluwer Health/Lippincott Williams & Wilkins; 2010.)

- Sonographic findings:
  ○ Bilateral enlarged kidneys with multiple renal cysts of varying sizes
  ○ Possible cysts within the liver, spleen, and/or pancreas
- Renal cell carcinoma (**Fig. 5-20**):
  - Clinical findings:
    - Hematuria
    - Weight loss
    - Palpable mass

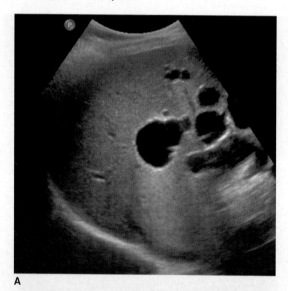

A

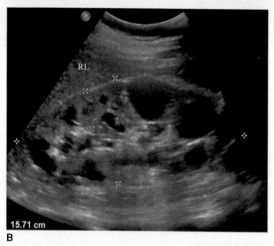

B

Figure 5-19. Renal and liver cysts. A: Multiple liver cysts are noted in this image of a patient with ADPKD. B: Multiple cysts are located throughout this kidney, which is indicative of ADPKD. (Reprinted with permission from Kawamura D, Lunsford B, eds. *Abdomen and Superficial Structures*. 3rd ed. Philadelphia, PA: Wolters Kluwer Health/Lippincott Williams & Wilkins; 2012.)

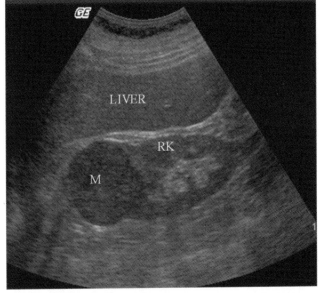

Figure 5-20. Renal cell carcinoma. A solid hypoechoic mass (*M*) is noted within the upper pole of this right kidney (*RK*) which is being imaged in the longitudinal plane. (Reprinted with permission from Kawamura D, Nolan T, eds. *Abdomen and Superficial Structures*. 4th ed. Philadelphia, PA: Wolters Kluwer; 2017.)

- Smoker
- Hypertension
- Flank pain
- Sonographic findings:
  - Hypoechoic, isoechoic, or hyperechoic solid mass on the kidney
  - Could appear as a complex cyst
  - Assess the renal vein and inferior vena cava (IVC) for possible tumor invasion
- Chronic renal failure (**Fig. 5-21**):
  - Clinical findings:
    - Diabetes
    - Malaise

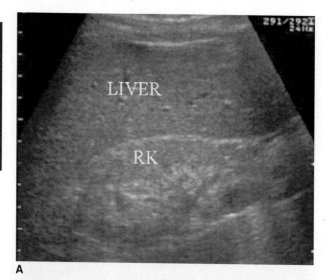

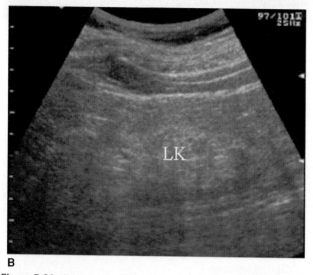

Figure 5-21. **Chronic renal failure. The right kidney (*RK*) (*A*) and the left kidney (*LK*) (*B*) are notably more echogenic than normal, indicating chronic renal failure.** (Images courtesy of Taco Geertsma, MD, Hospital Gelderse Vallei, Ede, The Netherlands.)

- Elevated BUN and creatinine
- Fatigue
- Hypertension
- Hyperkalemia (high levels of serum potassium)
- Sonographic findings:
  - Bilateral, small echogenic kidneys
  - Cortical thinning
  - Possible renal cysts
- Ureterocele—ballooning of the distal ureter into the bladder:
  - Clinical findings:
    - Asymptomatic
    - Urinary tract infection
  - Sonographic findings:
    - Anechoic, balloon-shaped structure within the lumen of the urinary bladder near the UVJ
- Cystitis—inflammation of the urinary bladder
  - Clinical findings:
    - Urinary tract infection
    - Pain in the bladder with urination
    - Hematuria
    - Dysuria
  - Sonographic findings:
    - Diffusely thickened urinary bladder wall measuring >4 mm in thickness
    - Perhaps some intraluminal, layering debris in bladder

WHERE ELSE TO LOOK

- An enlarged prostate can cause urinary symptom, so an assessment of the prostate transabdominally can be performed briefly in males.
- Don't forget to analyze the adrenal gland area in adults, because occasionally adrenal masses or cysts can be discovered sonographically.
- Large uterine or ovarian masses cause hydronephrosis and urinary symptoms.
- When a solid renal mass is identified, be sure to assess the IVC closely for signs of tumor invasion through the renal vein.

IMAGE CORRELATION

- Normal CT of the kidney **(Fig. 5-22)**
- Kidney stone on CT **(Fig. 5-23)**

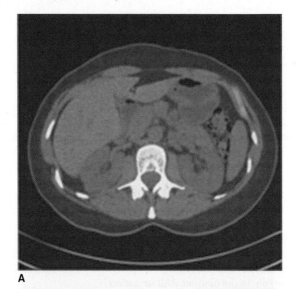

A

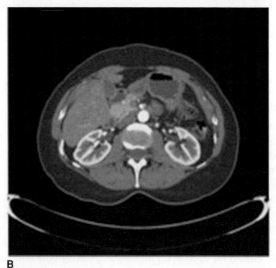

B

Figure 5-22. **Normal CT of the kidneys. A: Noncontrast image of the kidneys. B: Contrast image of the kidneys.** (Reprinted with permission from Smith WL, ed. *Radiology 101*. 4th ed. Philadelphia, PA: Wolters Kluwer Health/Lippincott Williams & Wilkins; 2013.)

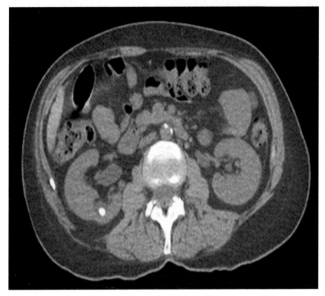

Figure 5-23. CT of kidney stone. A bright calcium stone is noted within the right kidney. (Reprinted with permission from Dunnick NR, Newhouse JH, Cohan RH, Maturen KE, eds. *Genitourinary Radiology.* 6th ed. Philadelphia, PA: Wolters Kluwer; 2017.)

REFERENCES

1. AIUM practice parameters for the performance of an ultrasound of the abdomen and/or retroperitoneum. http://www.aium.org/resources/guidelines/abdominal.pdf. Accessed October 14, 2018.
2. Penny SM. *Examination Review for Ultrasound: Abdomen & Obstetrics and Gynecology.* 2nd ed. Philadelphia, PA: Wolters Kluwer; 2018:107–136.
3. Sanders RC, Hall-Terracciano B. *Clinical Sonography: A Practical Guide.* 5th ed. Philadelphia, PA: Wolters Kluwer; 2016:421–435, 553–576, 596–604.
4. Seigel MJ. *Pediatric Sonography.* 4th ed. Philadelphia, PA: Wolters Kluwer; 2011:384–460.
5. Rumack CM, Wilson SR, Charboneau JW, Levine D. *Diagnostic Ultrasound.* 4th ed. Philadelphia, PA: Elsevier; 2011:317–391.

CHAPTER 6

Spleen

INTRODUCTION

The spleen, located in the left upper quadrant, may be a challenging organ to assess sonographically because of its normally small size. In some individuals, the problematic protecting ribs that lie adjacent to the spleen may offer only a sonographic glimpse at its form and structure. Nonetheless, the spleen should be evaluated systematically, especially if the patient has suffered from splenic trauma or if splenomegaly with associated portal hypertension is suspected clinically.

AIUM RECOMMENDATIONS FOR SONOGRAPHY OF THE SPLEEN[1]

- Assess the spleen in the following manner:
  - The spleen should be assessed for parenchymal abnormalities (e.g., masses, cysts, calcifications, etc.).
  - The echogenicity of the spleen should be compared to the left kidney when possible.
  - The left hemidiaphragm and the left pleural space should also be evaluated.

ESSENTIAL ANATOMY AND PHYSIOLOGY OF THE SPLEEN[2,3]

- The spleen is an intraperitoneal organ located in the left upper quadrant (Fig. 6-1).
- The spleen has a concave inferior surface and a convex superior surface and is about the size of the human fist.
- The splenic artery, which enters the spleen at the splenic hilum, is a branch of the celiac axis, a main branch of the abdominal aorta just above the superior mesenteric artery (Fig. 6-2).
- The splenic vein exits the splenic hilum and travels medially toward the pancreas, outlining the pancreatic tail posteriorly,

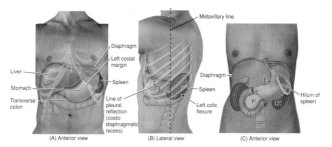

Figure 6-1. Location of the spleen. (Reprinted with permission from Moore KL, Dalley AF, Agur AM, eds. *Clinically Oriented Anatomy.* 6th ed. Philadelphia, PA: Wolters Kluwer Health/Lippincott Williams & Wilkins; 2009.)

ultimately continuing on to join with the inferior mesenteric vein and superior mesenteric vein to help create the main portal vein (Fig. 6-2).

- The spleen is the largest mass of lymphoid tissue in the body.
- The spleen acts as a center for erythropoiesis in the fetus and can revert to that function in adults. It is also a blood reservoir, it cleans or destroys defective red blood cells, and it acts in the immune response and thus is a protective organ against disease.

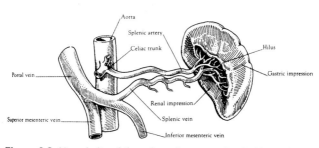

Figure 6-2. Vascularity of the spleen. (Images reprinted with permission from Kawamura D, ed. *Diagnostic Medical Sonography: Abdomen and Superficial Structures.* 2nd ed. Philadelphia, PA: Lippincott Williams & Wilkins; 1997:267.)

PATIENT PREPARATION FOR SONOGRAPHY OF THE SPLEEN

- Though fasting is often not necessary, it may be helpful in eliminating some adjacent bowel gas in some individuals, especially if the splenic hilum or splenic vasculature is of great interest.
- A distended stomach, which lies anterior to the spleen, could simulate pathology such as a pancreatic pseudocyst, so an inquiry should be performed as to the patient's fasting status.

SUGGESTED EQUIPMENT[3]

- 3.5–5-MHz transducer
- Higher frequencies can be used for thin patients and a small-footprint transducer may be required to visualize through narrow intercostal spaces
- General abdominal setting (most machines)
- Positional sponges for decubitus images

CLINICAL INVESTIGATION FOR SONOGRAPHY OF THE SPLEEN[2,3]

- Laboratory values are listed in Table 6.1.
- Evaluate prior imaging reports and images including CT, MRI, radiography, and any other appropriate tests.
- Critical clinical history questions related to the spleen[2]:
  - History of splenectomy? *Not only will the spleen be absent, but the motive for the previous splenectomy may be relevant.*
  - History of splenic or left upper quadrant trauma? *If the patient has a history of splenic trauma, there may be evidence of such trauma upon sonographic investigation,*

6. Spleen

Table 6-1	LAB FINDINGS AND POSSIBLE ASSOCIATED SPLENIC PATHOLOGY
LAB FINDING	POTENTIAL PATHOLOGY
↑ WBC (leukocytosis)	Inflammation, infection, hemorrhage, carcinoma, or acute leukemia
↓ WBC (leukopenia)	Radiation therapy, chemotherapy, lupus, vitamin B_{12} deficiency, viral infections, leukemia, and diabetes mellitus
↓ Hematocrit	Splenic hemorrhage

such as a notable laceration or hematoma. If trauma occurred long ago, calcifications may be present in the spleen representing a chronic hematoma.

- History of sickle cell anemia? *Sickle cell is most often found in African-American, Middle East, Mediterranean, and Hispanic children of Caribbean descent in the United States. Splenomegaly may be initially present, but with time the spleen can appear exceedingly irregular and can even waste away.*

NORMAL SONOGRAPHIC DESCRIPTION OF THE SPLEEN[2,3]

- The spleen is typically isoechoic to the normal liver, though it may be slightly more echogenic.
- The left kidney is normally more hypoechoic than the spleen.

SUGGESTED PROTOCOL FOR SONOGRAPHY OF THE SPLEEN

- Survey the spleen in transverse or longitudinal:
  - Ask the patient to extend his or her left arm up above his or her head in order to expand the intercostal spaces.
  - With the patient in the supine position, obtain a brief survey of the spleen by scanning superiorly and inferiorly (transverse) or anterior to posterior (longitudinal).
  - Obtain a brief video clip of the spleen in longitudinal and transverse **(Video 6-1 and Video 6-2)**.
- Longitudinal spleen **(Fig. 6-3)**:
  - Supine interrogation may be helpful for some patients, though the right lateral decubitus position is most often employed.
  - Transducer placement is typically along the left midaxillary line, between the intercostal spaces, which results in a coronal section of the spleen (often labeled longitudinal or sagittal).
  - The index or notch on the transducer may need to be tilted or angled slightly posteriorly to obtain the entire length of the spleen **(Fig. 6-4)**.
  - Deep inspiration results in inferiorly displacing the spleen. Conversely, complete expiration may be helpful with some patients.
  - An attempt to visualize both the superior and inferior aspects of the spleen should be made.

6. Spleen

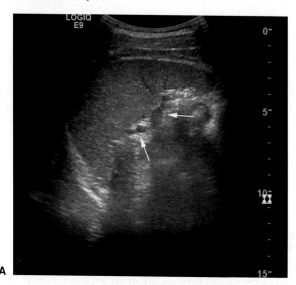

A

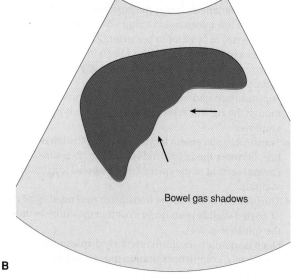

B

Figure 6-3. Longitudinal spleen. A, B: Longitudinal spleen at the level of the splenic hilum (*arrows*). (Image A courtesy of Philips Medical System, Bothell, WA.)

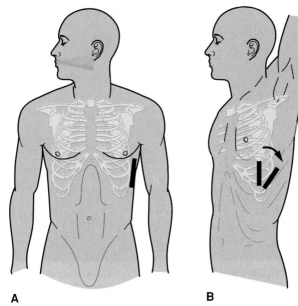

A   **B**

Figure 6-4. Transducer placement for longitudinal spleen images.
**A: Transducer placement is typically along the left midaxillary line,
between the intercostal spaces, which results in a coronal section
of the spleen (often labeled longitudinal or sagittal). B: The index
or notch on the transducer may need to be tilted or angled slightly
posteriorly to obtain the entire length of the spleen.** (Reprinted with
permission from Cosby KS, Kendall JL, eds. *Practical Guide to Emergency
Ultrasound.* 2nd ed. Philadelphia, PA: Wolters Kluwer Health/Lippincott
Williams & Wilkins; 2013.)

- Several images may be needed to completely demonstrate
  the sagittal spleen.
- The spleen can be scanned completely by angling or
  manipulating the transducer through the intercostal spaces
  from anterior to posterior.
- The spleen should be uniform in echogenicity, though
  occasionally small, anechoic blood vessels may be noted
  within the parenchyma and can be thus proven to be
  vascular structures with color Doppler.
- An evaluation of the spleen for solid masses, cysts, and
  adjacent fluid collections and lacerations or hematomas
  should be performed when trauma has occurred.

6. Spleen

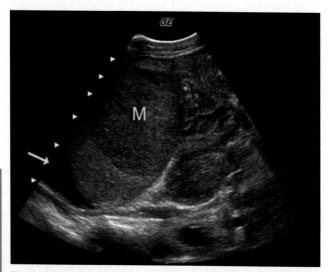

Figure 6-5. Left-sided pleural effusion. An anechoic fluid collection (*arrow*) above the diaphragm in this patient, representing a pleural effusion. This patient also has a splenic mass (*M*). (Reprinted with permission from Layon AJ, Gabrielli A, Yu M, Wood KE, eds. *Civetta, Taylor, & Kirby's Critical Care Medicine.* 5th ed. Philadelphia, PA: Wolters Kluwer; 2017.)

- - The right hemidiaphragm should be assessed for signs of pleural fluid (**Fig. 6-5**).
  - If required, a longitudinal measurement of the spleen can be obtained (**Fig. 6-6**).
- Transverse spleen (**Fig. 6-7**):
  - Supine interrogation may be helpful for some patients, though the right lateral decubitus position is most often employed.
  - The transducer should be placed in an orthogonal plane (90°) to the longitudinal image obtained.
  - The spleen should be scanned completely from superior to inferior in the transverse plane.
  - The spleen should be uniform in echogenicity, though occasionally small, anechoic blood vessels may be noted within the parenchyma and can be thus proven to be vascular structures with color Doppler.

6. Spleen

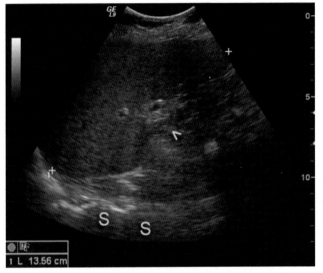

Figure 6-6. Longitudinal spleen with measurement. Longitudinal measurement of the spleen (between *calipers*) at the level of the midaxillary line demonstrating the splenic hilum (*arrowhead*). The spleen measures upper limits of normal. The spine (*S*) can also be seen. (Reprinted with permission from Sanders RC, eds. *Clinical Sonography: A Practical Guide.* 5th ed. Philadelphia, PA: Wolters Kluwer; 2015.)

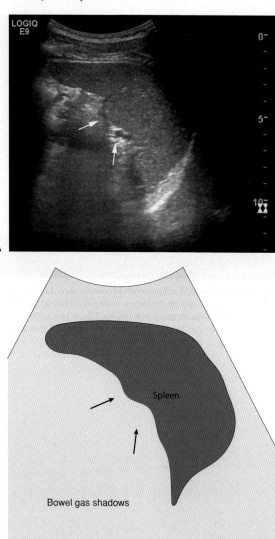

Figure 6-7. Transverse image of the spleen. A, B: Transverse image of the spleen at the level of the splenic hilum (*arrows*). (Reprinted with permission from Erkonen WE, Smith WL, eds. *Radiology 101*. 2nd ed. Philadelphia, PA: Lippincott Williams & Wilkins; 2004.)

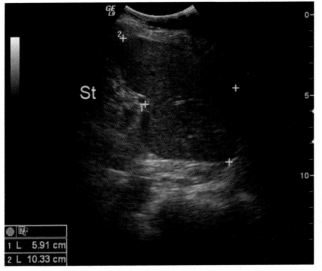

Figure 6-8. Transverse spleen with measurement. Transverse measurements of the spleen (between *calipers*). This spleen measured upper limits of normal in the longitudinal plane demonstrated in Figure 6-6. The area of the stomach (*ST*) can also be seen. (Reprinted with permission from Sanders RC, ed. *Clinical Sonography: A Practical Guide.* 5th ed. Philadelphia, PA: Wolters Kluwer; 2015.)

- The spleen should be evaluated for solid masses, cysts, and adjacent fluid collections and lacerations or hematomas when trauma has occurred.
- The left hemidiaphragm should be assessed for signs of pleural fluid.
- If required, a longitudinal measurement of the spleen can be obtained (Fig. 6-8).
- Additional images:
  - Longitudinal or transverse splenic hilum with color Doppler (Fig. 6-9):
    - Longitudinal orientation may require angling the transducer slightly anterior to see the medially positioned splenic hilum.
    - This image is useful when analyzing the splenic hilum for signs of dilated varicosities associated with splenomegaly and portal hypertension.

6. Spleen

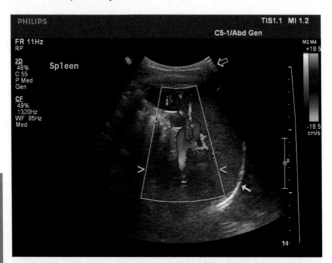

Figure 6-9. Color Doppler of the splenic hilum. This transverse view of the spleen was taken with the patient supine. The color box has been reduced to the area of the splenic hilum (*arrowheads*). The curvilinear diaphragm appears as an echogenic structure (*arrow*). A rib produces a reverberation artifact and shadowing (*open arrow*). The splenic vein is demonstrated by the large blue-colored structure in the center of the splenic hilum and the color box. (Reprinted with permission from Sanders RC, ed. *Clinical Sonography: A Practical Guide.* 5th ed. Philadelphia, PA: Wolters Kluwer; 2015.)

SCANNING TIPS

- Don't be too quick to place the patient in right lateral decubitus position, because in some individuals the spleen may be evaluated better in the supine position.
- Occasionally, the spleen of thin or pediatric patients may be assessed from posterior, through the back musculature.
- In the right lateral decubitus position, for patients with a large disparity between the waste and the hips, place a positioning sponge or pillow under the patient's right side to lessen the disproportion.
- Some patients may have an accessory spleen, most likely located in the area of the splenic hilum (**Fig. 6-10**).
- Splenomegaly is often suspected sonographically if the spleen extends beyond the inferior pole of the left kidney in the sagittal plane.

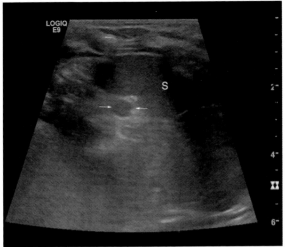

A

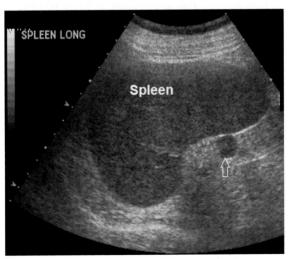

B

Figure 6-10. **Accessory spleen. Transverse (A) and longitudinal (B) images of the spleen (S) with an adjacent accessory spleen (arrows) noted in the area of the splenic hilum.** (Reprinted with permission from Sanders RC, ed. *Clinical Sonography: A Practical Guide.* 5th ed. Philadelphia, PA: Wolters Kluwer; 2015.)

- Lymphoma and leukemia may manifest as splenomegaly or focal masses may be identified.

NORMAL MEASUREMENTS OF THE SPLEEN[*3]

- Length = 12–13 cm
- Anteroposterior = <8 cm
- Transverse dimension = <4 cm

ESSENTIAL SPLENIC PATHOLOGY[2]

- Splenomegaly—enlargement of the spleen (Fig. 6-11):
  - Clinical findings:
    - Palpable, enlarged spleen
    - History of cirrhosis, leukemia, or lymphoma
    - Hemolytic abnormality like sickle cell
    - Trauma
    - Infection
    - Elevated WBC and/or red blood cell count
  - Sonographic findings:
    - Enlargement of the spleen based on measurements
    - Spleen notably extends beyond the inferior pole of the left kidney in sagittal
- Splenic trauma—the spleen is often injured in cases of blunt trauma (Fig. 6-12):
  - Clinical findings:
    - Blunt trauma to the left upper quadrant
    - Left upper quadrant pain
    - Possible decreased hematocrit
  - Sonographic findings:
    - Evidence of hemorrhage may be found within and/or around the spleen
    - Acute hemorrhagic stage—complex or hypoechoic
    - Middle stage—echogenic or isoechoic
    - Later stage—anechoic or hypoechoic
    - Chronic stage—complex appearance and may have calcified components

---

*Women typically have a smaller spleen than men, and the spleen often decreases in size with advancing age.

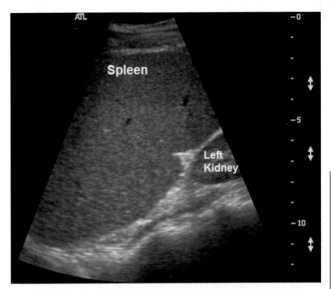

Figure 6-11. Splenomegaly. In the sagittal plane, this spleen is notable large in comparison to the left kidney. (Reprinted with permission from Kawamura D, Nolan T, eds. *Abdomen and Superficial Structures*. 4th ed. Philadelphia, PA: Wolters Kluwer; 2017.)

6. Spleen

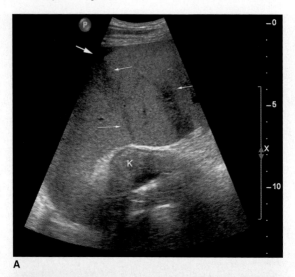

A

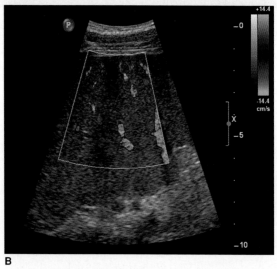

B

Figure 6-12. Splenic trauma and rupture. A: Longitudinal image of a ruptured spleen with a notable laceration (*small arrows*) and blood adjacent to the spleen (*larger arrow*). B: Transverse image of the same patient with color Doppler applied. Note that splenomegaly is also evident on these images. (Images courtesy of Philips Medical System, Bothell, WA.)

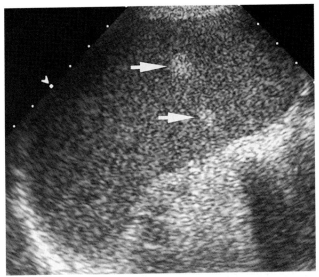

Figure 6-13. Splenic hemangioma. Two hyperechoic masses (*arrows*) are noted within this spleen. (Reprinted with permission from Siegel MJ, Coley B, eds. *Core Curriculum: Pediatric Imaging.* Philadelphia, PA: Lippincott Williams & Wilkins; 2005.)

- Hemangioma—a common benign mass of the spleen that consists of blood vessels **(Fig. 6-13)**:
  - Clinical findings:
    - Asymptomatic
  - Sonographic findings:
    - Hyperechoic mass
- Splenic infarct—tissue death to a portion of the spleen that results from the deprivation of oxygen **(Fig. 6-14)**:
  - Clinical findings:
    - Patient may have sudden onset of left upper quadrant pain.
    - Patient may be suffering from sickle cell anemia, bacterial endocarditis, vasculitis, or lymphoma.
  - Sonographic findings:
    - Acute infarct—hypoechoic, wedge-shaped mass within the spleen
    - Chronic infarct—hyperechoic, wedge-shaped mass within the spleen

6. Spleen

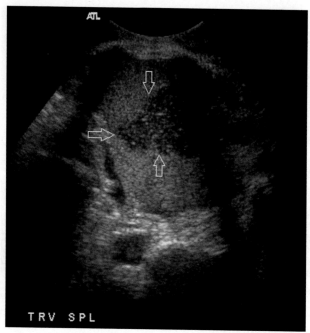

Figure 6-14. Splenic infarct. A hypoechoic, wedge-shaped mass
(between *arrows*) **is noted within this spleen representing a splenic
infarct.** (Reprinted with permission from Kawamura D, Nolan T, eds. *Abdomen
and Superficial Structures*. 4th ed. Philadelphia, PA: Wolters Kluwer; 2017.)

WHERE ELSE TO LOOK[2]

- Children with sickle cell anemia are prone to develop
  gallstones, so a thorough assessment of the gallbladder may
  be reasonable.
- Implantations of ectopic splenic tissue can be the result of
  splenic rupture, a condition referred to as splenosis. These
  implants can be dispersed throughout the abdomen and
  can simulate solid masses. Clinical evaluation is vital for the
  diagnosis of this condition.

IMAGE CORRELATION

- Normal spleen on CT (Fig. 6-15)
- Splenomegaly on CT (Fig. 6-16)
- Splenic trauma on CT (Fig. 6-17)

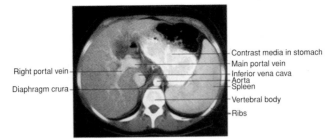

Figure 6-15. CT of a normal spleen. (Reprinted with permission from Smith WL, ed. *Radiology 101*. 4th ed. Philadelphia, PA: Wolters Kluwer Health/Lippincott Williams & Wilkins; 2013.)

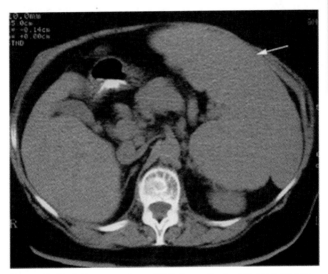

Figure 6-16. Splenomegaly on CT. A dramatically enlarged spleen (*arrow*) is noted on the CT image of the abdomen. (Reprinted with permission from Silberman H, Silberman AW, eds. *Principles and Practice of Surgical Oncology*. Philadelphia, PA: Wolters Kluwer Health/Lippincott Williams & Wilkins; 2009.)

6. Spleen

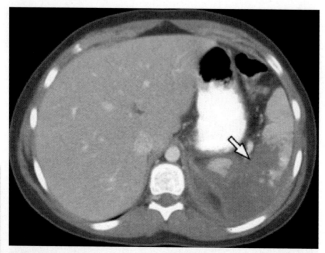

Figure 6-17. Splenic trauma on CT. Splenic trauma in a 12-year-old girl after a snowboarding accident. Axial contrast-enhanced CT image shows a large splenic laceration (*arrow*) with devascularization of a portion of the splenic parenchyma. (Reprinted with permission from Lee E, ed. *Pediatric Radiology: Practical Imaging Evaluation of Infants and Children.* Philadelphia, PA: Wolters Kluwer; 2017.)

REFERENCES

1. AIUM practice parameters for the performance of an ultrasound of the abdomen and/or retroperitoneum. http://www.aium.org/resources/guidelines/abdominal.pdf. Accessed June 27, 2018.
2. Penny SM. *Examination Review for Ultrasound: Abdomen & Obstetrics and Gynecology.* 2nd ed. Philadelphia, PA: Wolters Kluwer; 2018:1–78.
3. Kawamura DM, Nolan TD. *Diagnostic Medical Sonography: Abdomen and Superficial Structures.* 4th ed. Philadelphia, PA: Wolters Kluwer; 2018: 171–212.

CHAPTER 7

Abdominal Aorta and Inferior Vena Cava

INTRODUCTION

This chapter will provide a sonographic protocol for imaging of the abdominal aorta and inferior vena cava (IVC). Also, vasculature assessment of the various branches of the abdominal aorta and IVC will be provided. However, assessment of the portal venous system can be found in Chapter 3, while the evaluation of renal vasculature is mentioned in this chapter and further information can be found in Chapter 5.

AIUM RECOMMENDATIONS FOR SONOGRAPHY OF THE ABDOMINAL AORTA AND IVC

- Assess the abdominal aorta and IVC in the following manner:
  - The abdominal aorta should be examined when there is a palpable or pulsatile abdominal mass or bruit.
  - The abdominal aorta should be examined when there is unexplained lower back pain, flank pain, or abdominal pain.
  - The abdominal aorta should be examined as a follow-up of previously demonstrated abdominal aortic aneurysm (AAA) or to assess a previously instilled abdominal aortic and/or iliac endoluminal stent graft.
  - The IVC should be evaluated for abnormalities, patency, vena cava filters, interruption devices, and catheters and their location in respect to the hepatic veins and/or renal veins.

ESSENTIAL ANATOMY AND PHYSIOLOGY OF THE ABDOMINAL AORTA AND IVC

- Abdominal aorta:
  - The aorta originates at the left ventricle of the heart (Fig. 7-1).

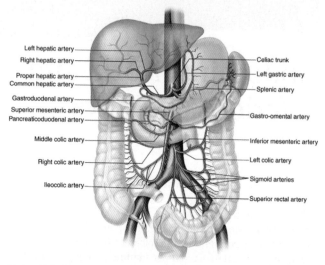

Figure 7-1. Anatomy of the abdominal aorta and its branches.
(Reprinted with permission from Kupinski AM, ed. *The Vascular System.*
2nd ed. Philadelphia, PA: Wolters Kluwer; 2017.)

- The abdominal aorta, which is the largest artery in the abdomen, is located just left of the midline within the retroperitoneum.
- The abdominal aorta tapers as it travels inferiorly from the diaphragm.
- The major branches of the abdominal aorta from superior to inferior include the following:
  - Celiac artery:
    - The celiac artery, also referred to as the celiac trunk or celiac axis, branches into the common hepatic artery, splenic artery, and left gastric artery.
  - Superior mesenteric artery
  - Renal arteries (right and left)
  - Inferior mesenteric artery
  - Common iliac arteries (right and left)
    - Also referred to as the aortic bifurcation
- The function of the abdominal aorta is to provide oxygenated blood to the abdomen, pelvis, and lower extremities.

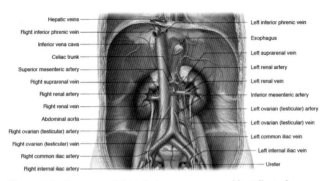

Hepatic veins
Right inferior phrenic vein
Inferior vena cava
Celiac trunk
Superior mesenteric artery
Right suprarenal vein
Right renal artery
Right renal vein
Abdominal aorta
Right ovarian (testicular) artery
Right ovarian (testicular) vein
Right common iliac artery
Right internal iliac artery

Left inferior phrenic vein
Esophagus
Left suprarenal vein
Left renal artery
Left renal vein
Inferior mesenteric artery
Left ovarian (testicular) artery
Left ovarian (testicular) vein
Left common iliac vein
Left internal iliac vein
Ureter

Figure 7-2. Anatomy of the inferior vena cava and its tributaries.
(Reprinted with permission from Kupinski AM, ed. *The Vascular System.*
Philadelphia, PA: Wolters Kluwer Health/Lippincott Williams & Wilkins; 2012.)

- IVC:
  - The IVC is created by the union of the two common iliac veins **(Fig. 7-2)**.
  - The IVC travels cephalad, coursing through the abdomen right lateral to the aorta and posterior to the liver.
  - The IVC terminates at the right atrium.
  - The major veins that drain into the IVC from superior to inferior include the following:
    - Hepatic veins (right, middle, and left)
    - Renal veins (right and left)
    - Common iliac veins (right and left)
  - The primary function of the IVC is to return blood from the abdomen back to the heart.

PATIENT PREPARATION FOR SONOGRAPHY OF THE ABDOMINAL AORTA AND IVC[1]

- Fasting for 8–12 hrs for a sonogram of the abdominal aorta and IVC commensurate with a complete abdomen examination would be optimal, though emergency sonograms may need to be immediately performed without patient preparation.

SUGGESTED EQUIPMENT[1,2]

- Some machines may have abdominal aorta settings, while others may suggest the general abdominal setting.

- For adults, mean frequencies between 4 and 6 MHz are most commonly used.
- However, for patients with increased abdominal girth lower frequencies may be warranted for better penetration.

CLINICAL INVESTIGATION FOR SONOGRAPHY OF THE ABDOMINAL AORTA AND IVC

- Laboratory values are listed in **Table 7-1**.
- Evaluate prior imaging reports and images including CT, MRI, radiography, and any other appropriate tests.
- Critical clinical history questions related to the abdominal aorta and IVC:
  - Do you have a history of smoking or atherosclerosis? *Patients who smoke or who have atherosclerosis are at increased risk for thrombosis and AAAs.*
  - Do you have pain in the legs, hip, or buttocks after exercise (This is referred to as claudication and it is secondary to decreased blood supply)? *Claudication can be a sign of vascular obstruction, peripheral artery disease, and aneurismal involvement of the abdominal aorta or iliac arteries.*
  - Do you have back and/or chest pain? *Back and/or chest pain is a symptom of aneurysms and rupture.*
  - Do you have pain at rest in your limbs? *This is a sign of ischemic rest pain and it is associated with vascular compromise to the extremities which may be associated with an aneurysm.*
  - History of abdominal surgery or AAA repair? *This is important information to have before beginning the examination. Any pertinent history, such as the preoperative size of the aneurysm and the type and date of repair is most beneficial.*

Table 7-1	LAB FINDINGS AND POSSIBLE ASSOCIATED AORTIC PATHOLOGY

LAB FINDING	POTENTIAL PATHOLOGY
↑ WBC (leukocytosis)	Inflammation, infection, hemorrhage, or carcinoma
↓ Hematocrit	Aortic rupture

NORMAL SONOGRAPHIC DESCRIPTION OF THE ABDOMINAL AORTA AND IVC

- Abdominal aorta:
  - The abdominal aorta appears as an anechoic tube that begins below the diaphragm and extends down to the umbilicus, where it bifurcates into the common iliac arteries.
  - The abdominal aorta is located anterior to the spine and just left of the midline.
- IVC:
  - The abdominal portion of the IVC appears as an anechoic tube that travels from the diaphragm on the right side, just behind the liver, to the umbilicus where the common iliac veins join.
  - The diameter of the IVC can vary with respiration. Suspending respiration will initially cause the IVC to reduce in diameter, while prolonged suspension of respirations will cause the IVC to increase in diameter.

SUGGESTED PROTOCOL FOR SONOGRAPHY OF THE ABDOMINAL AORTA AND IVC[2]

- Survey the abdominal aorta in longitudinal or transverse:
  - With the patient in the supine position, obtain a brief survey of the abdominal aorta by scanning superior to inferior in longitudinal or transverse.
  - Assess the abdominal aorta for focal enlargement and intraluminal abnormalities.
  - Obtain a brief video clip of the abdominal aorta **(Video 7-1).** ▶️
- Longitudinal proximal aorta:
  - Image the proximal abdominal aorta along the long axis of the lumen of the vessel.
  - Demonstrate the celiac axis and superior mesenteric artery.
  - Obtain images with and without an anteroposterior measurement of the proximal abdominal aorta from the outer edge to outer edge **(Fig. 7-3).**
  - If an AAA is present, document and record the maximal size and location of the aneurysm. The relationship of the dilated segment to the renal arteries and to the aortic bifurcation should be determined if possible.

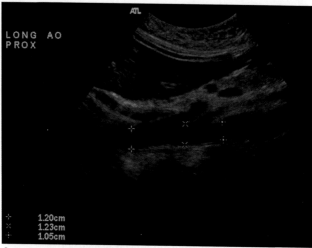

A

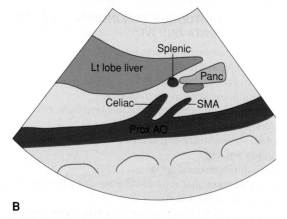

B

Figure 7-3. **Longitudinal proximal abdominal aorta with measurement. A, B: Longitudinal image of the proximal aorta (Prox AO), including the celiac artery (Celiac), superior mesenteric artery (SMA), splenic artery (Splenic), pancreas (Panc), and left lobe of the liver (Lt lobe liver).**

- Longitudinal mid aorta:
  - Image the mid abdominal aorta along the long axis of the lumen of the vessel.
  - Demonstrate the level of the renal arteries.
  - Obtain images with and without an anteroposterior measurement of the mid abdominal aorta from the outer edge to outer edge **(Fig. 7-4)**.
  - If an AAA is present, document and record the maximal size and location of the aneurysm. The relationship of the dilated segment to the renal arteries and to the aortic bifurcation should be determined if possible.
- Longitudinal distal aorta:
  - Image the distal abdominal aorta along the long axis of the vessel.
  - Demonstrate the distal aorta above the iliac bifurcation.
  - Obtain images with and without a measurement of the distal abdominal aorta from the anterior outer edge to outer edge **(Fig. 7-5)**.
  - If an AAA is present, document and record the maximal size and location of the aneurysm. The relationship of the dilated segment to the renal arteries and to the aortic bifurcation should be determined if possible.
- Transverse proximal abdominal aorta:
  - Image the proximal abdominal aorta perpendicular to the long axis of the vessel **(Fig. 7-6)**.
  - Demonstrate the abdominal aorta below the diaphragm, near the celiac axis.
  - Obtain images with and without a width measurement of the proximal abdominal aorta from the outer edge to outer edge.
  - If an AAA is present, document and record the maximal size and location of the aneurysm. The relationship of the dilated segment to the renal arteries and to the aortic bifurcation should be determined if possible.
- Transverse mid aorta:
  - Image the mid abdominal aorta perpendicular to the long axis of the vessel.
  - Demonstrate the level of the renal arteries **(Fig. 7-7)**.
  - Obtain images with and without a width measurement of the mid abdominal aorta from the outer edge to outer edge.

7. Abdominal Aorta

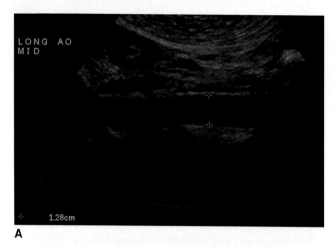

A

B

Figure 7-4. **Longitudinal mid abdominal aorta with measurement.**
A,B: Longitudinal mid abdominal aorta with measurement.

7. Abdominal Aorta

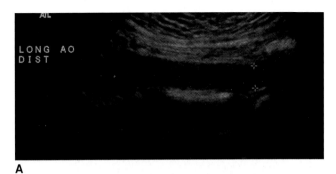

A

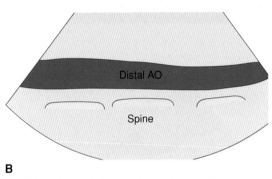

B

Figure 7-5. **Longitudinal distal abdominal aorta with measurement.**
A,B: Longitudinal image of the distal aorta with measurement
obtained just proximal to the bifurcation.

7. Abdominal Aorta

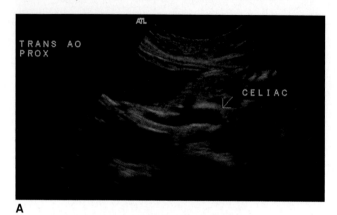

A

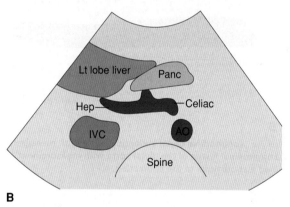

B

7. Abdominal Aorta

Figure 7-6. **Transverse proximal celiac level. A,B: Transverse image of the proximal aorta (AO) at the level of the celiac artery (Celiac). Also noted are the spine, inferior vena cava (IVC), hepatic artery (Hep), left lobe of the liver (Lt lobe liver), and the pancreas (Panc).**

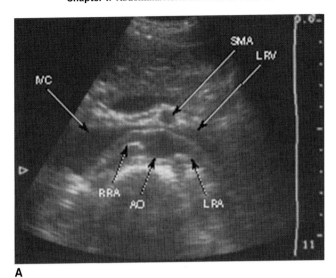

A

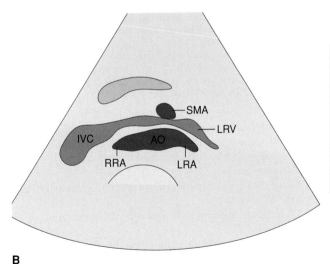

B

Figure 7-7. Transverse mid abdominal aorta renal level with measurement. A,B: Transverse at the level of the renal vessels. *(continued)*

7. Abdominal Aorta

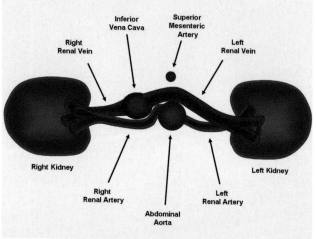

C

Figure 7-7 *(continued)*. **C: Diagram of the typical orientation of the renal vessel in transverse. AO, aorta; IVC, inferior vena cava; LRA, left renal artery; LRV, left renal vein; RRA, right renal artery; SMA, superior mesenteric artery.** (Part A reprinted with permission from Cosby K, Kendall J, eds. *Practical Guide to Emergency Ultrasound.* Philadelphia, PA: Lippincott Williams & Wilkins; 2006:227. Part C reprinted with permission from Zierler RE, Dawson DL, eds. *Strandness's Duplex Scanning in Vascular Disorders.* 5th ed. Philadelphia, PA: Wolters Kluwer; 2015.)

- If an AAA is present, document and record the maximal size and location of the aneurysm. The relationship of the dilated segment to the renal arteries and to the aortic bifurcation should be determined if possible.
- Transverse distal aorta:
  - Image the distal abdominal aorta perpendicular to the long axis of the vessel.
  - Demonstrate the aorta just above the iliac bifurcation (Fig. 7-8).
  - Obtain images with and without a width measurement of the distal abdominal aorta from the outer edge to outer edge.
  - If an AAA is present, document and record the maximal size and location of the aneurysm. The relationship of the dilated segment to the renal arteries and to the aortic bifurcation should be determined if possible.

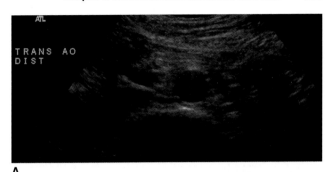

A

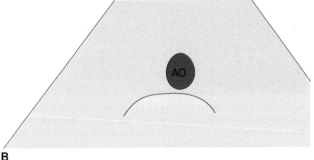

B

Figure 7-8. **Transverse distal abdominal aorta. A,B: Transverse image of the abdominal aorta (AO) just proximal to the aortic bifurcation.**

- Common iliac arteries:
  - Longitudinal images of the proximal right and left common iliac arteries should be obtained. These images should be obtained along the long axis of each vessel (**Fig. 7-9**).
  - Transverse images of the proximal right and left common iliac arteries should be obtained. These images should be obtained perpendicular to the long axis of each vessel (**Fig. 7-10**).
  - Measurement of the widest portion of each common iliac artery should be obtained from outer edge to outer edge.
  - If an iliac artery aneurysm is present, the maximal size and location of the aneurysm should be documented and recorded.

7. Abdominal Aorta

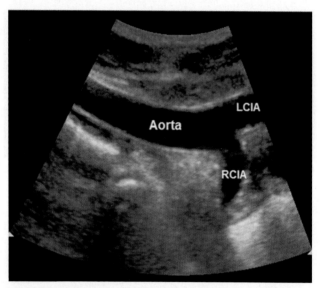

Figure 7-9. Longitudinal oblique image of the proximal common iliac arteries. This image demonstrates the distal aorta with the bifurcation, including both the left common iliac artery (LCIA) and right common iliac artery (RCIA). (Image courtesy of Philips Medical System, Bothell, WA.)

- Longitudinal and transverse IVC:
  - The hepatic section of the IVC can be demonstrated in longitudinal.
  - The renal section of the IVC can be demonstrated in the longitudinal and transverse plane (Fig. 7-11).
  - The infrarenal section of the IVC can be demonstrated in the longitudinal and transverse plane.
- Additional images[1,3]:
  - Color Doppler and/or spectral Doppler imaging with waveform analysis of the aorta and iliac arteries may be helpful to demonstrate patency and the presence of intraluminal thrombus.
    - Suprarenal aorta = low-resistance flow (Fig. 7-12)
    - Infrarenal aorta = high-resistance flow (Fig. 7-13)
  - Some facilities may require an additional assessment of the kidneys when the abdominal aorta is being examined and vice versa.

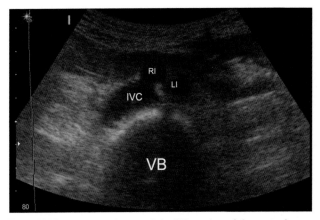

Figure 7-10. Transverse image of the bifurcation of the aorta. In this image, the right iliac artery (RI) and left iliac artery (LI) are seen slightly anterior to the inferior vena cava (IVC) and distal vertebral body (VB). (Reprinted with permission from Cosby KS, Kendall JL, eds. *Practical Guide to Emergency Ultrasound.* 2nd ed. Philadelphia, PA: Wolters Kluwer Health/Lippincott Williams & Wilkins; 2013.)

- Extended field of view, dual imaging, and landscape images can provide further documentation as to the relationship of an AAA.
- A Doppler assessment of the main branches of the abdominal aorta may be performed[1,3]:
  - Celiac artery = low-resistance flow:
    - Common hepatic artery = low-resistance flow
    - Splenic artery = low-resistance flow
  - Superior mesenteric artery:
    - Fasting patient = high-resistance flow **(Fig. 7-14)**
    - 30–90 min postprandial = low-resistance flow
  - Renal arteries = low-resistance flow
  - Common Iliac arteries = high-resistance flow
- Color Doppler and/or spectral Doppler imaging with waveform analysis of the IVC may be helpful to demonstrate patency and the presence of intraluminal thrombus.
  - IVC = pulsatile near the heart and more phasic near the common iliac veins **(Fig. 7-15)**
  - Hepatic veins = pulsatile, triphasic flow pattern
  - Renal veins = low-velocity, continuous flow

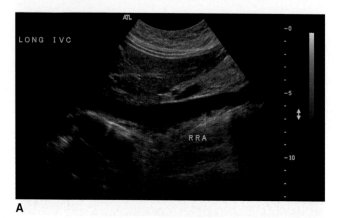

A

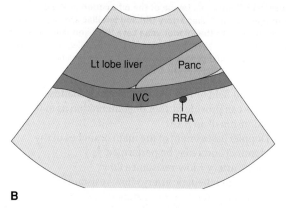

B

Figure 7-11. **Longitudinal image of the inferior vena cava.**
A,B: Longitudinal image of the inferior vena cava (IVC). Also
demonstrated are the left lobe of the liver, pancreas (PANC), and
right renal artery (RRA), which is located posterior to the IVC.

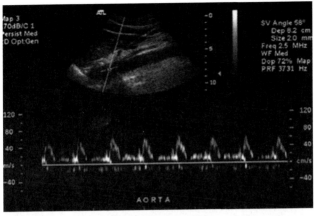

Figure 7-12. Low-resistance spectral waveform superior to the celiac artery. (Reprinted with permission from Kupinski AM, ed. *The Vascular System*. Philadelphia, PA: Wolters Kluwer Health/Lippincott Williams & Wilkins; 2012.)

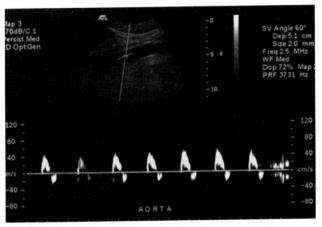

Figure 7-13. Higher-resistance spectral waveform in the distal aorta. (Reprinted with permission from Kupinski AM, ed. *The Vascular System*. 2nd ed. Philadelphia, PA: Wolters Kluwer; 2017.)

7. Abdominal Aorta

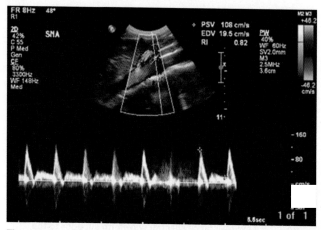

Figure 7-14. Normal high-resistance flow of the superior mesenteric artery. (Reprinted with permission from Kupinski AM, ed. *The Vascular System*. 2nd ed. Philadelphia, PA: Wolters Kluwer; 2017.)

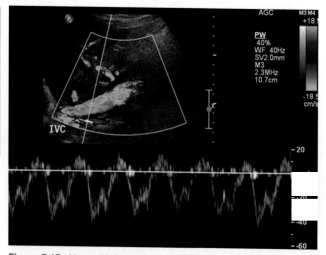

Figure 7-15. **Normal inferior vena cava Doppler analysis. The flow within the IVC demonstrates slight pulsatility caused by the proximity of the heart.** (Reprinted with permission from Kupinski AM, ed. *The Vascular System*. 2nd ed. Philadelphia, PA: Wolters Kluwer; 2017.)

SCANNING TIPS[4,5]

- Deep inspiration or complete expiration may assist in visualizing parts of the abdominal aorta.
- Scanning from the left flank, with the patient in the left lateral decubitus position, may assist in the visualization of the middle to distal abdominal aorta in obese patients.

NORMAL MEASUREMENTS OF THE ABDOMINAL AORTA AND IVC[1,3–5]

- Abdominal aorta:
  - Supraceliac = 2.5–2.7 cm in men and 2.1–2.3 cm in women
  - Infrarenal = 2.0–2.4 cm in men and 1.7–2.2 cm in women
  - Common iliac arteries = <1.5 cm
- IVC:
  - 2.5 cm or less

ESSENTIAL ABDOMINAL AORTA AND IVC PATHOLOGY[3]

- AAA—enlargement of the abdominal aorta:
  - Clinical findings:
    - Pulsatile abdominal mass
    - Abdominal bruit
    - Back pain
    - Abdominal pain
    - Lower-extremity pain (claudication)
  - Sonographic findings:
    - Diameter of the aorta measures >3 cm **(Fig. 7-16)**.
    - Thrombus is found within the aorta.
    - Old thrombus may calcify and shadow.
    - Most AAAs are located infrarenal and many involve the common iliac arteries.
    - Most AAAs are fusiform, which is a gradual enlargement of the abdominal aorta.
- Abdominal aortic dissection—separation of the layers of the wall of the abdominal aorta
  - Clinical findings:
    - Intense chest pain
    - Hypertension
    - Abdominal pain
    - Lower back pain
    - Neurologic symptoms

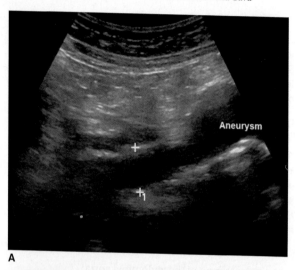

A

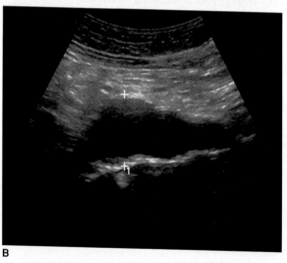

B

Figure 7-16. Abdominal aortic aneurysm. A: Normal aortic diameter (between *calipers*) with an aneurysm visualized distally. B: An abdominal aortic aneurysm is noted (between *calipers*).
(Reprinted with permission from Kawamura D, Lunsford B, eds. *Abdomen and Superficial Structures*. 3rd ed. Philadelphia, PA: Wolters Kluwer Health/ Lippincott Williams & Wilkins; 2012.)

- Sonographic findings:
  - Possible AAA
  - Intimal flap may be noted **(Fig. 7-17)**
- IVC thrombosis—clot within the IVC:
  - Clinical findings:
    - History of venous thrombus and blood clotting issues

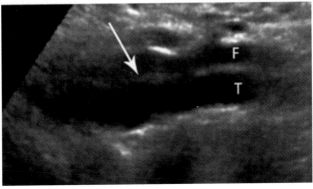

A

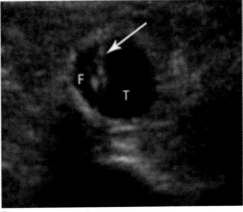

B

Figure 7-17. **Aortic dissection. A,B: An intimal flap (*arrow*) is noted in the presence of an aortic dissection, which also has a true (T) and false (F) lumen.** (Reprinted with permission from Brant WE, Helms C, eds. *Fundamentals of Diagnostic Radiology.* 4th ed. Philadelphia, PA: Wolters Kluwer Health/Lippincott Williams & Wilkins; 2012.)

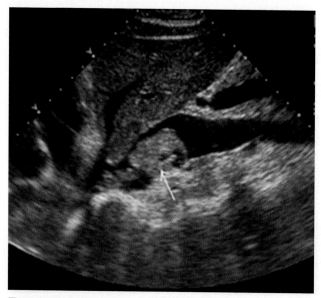

Figure 7-18. Inferior vena cava thrombus. Thrombus is noted with the inferior vena cava (*arrow*). (Reprinted with permission from Penny SM, ed. *Examination Review for Ultrasound*. Philadelphia, PA: Wolters Kluwer Health/Lippincott Williams & Wilkins; 2010.)

- Sonographic findings:
  - Hyperechoic clot within the lumen of the IVC **(Fig. 7-18)**
  - Thrombus may be isoechoic to surrounding blood
  - Present, diminished, or absent flow (occluded) within the IVC

WHERE ELSE TO LOOK

- Often, the kidneys need to be evaluated in relationship to an AAA. Assess vascular compromise to the kidneys by evaluating the main renal arteries and their branches and renal veins.
- When an AAA is noted, evaluate associated enlargement of the common iliac arteries.

IMAGE CORRELATION

- AAA on CT **(Fig. 7-19)**
- AAA on MRI **(Fig. 7-20)**

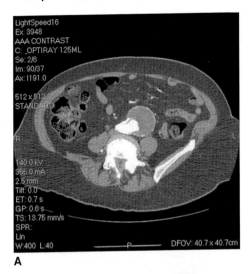

A

B

Figure 7-19. Computed tomography of an AAA. A: Typical appearance of an AAA on CT. B: Computed tomography angiogram image of an AAA. (Reprinted with permission from Madden M, ed. *Introduction to Sectional Anatomy.* 3rd ed. Philadelphia, PA: Wolters Kluwer Health/Lippincott Williams & Wilkins; 2012.)

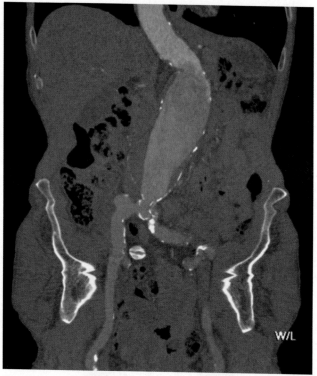

Figure 7-20. MRI coronal image of an AAA. (Reprinted with permission from Higgins CB, de Roos A, eds. *MRI and CT of the Cardiovascular System.* 3rd ed. Philadelphia, PA: Wolters Kluwer Health/Lippincott Williams & Wilkins; 2013.)

REFERENCES

1. Kupinski AM. *The Vascular System*. 2nd ed. Philadelphia, PA: Wolters Kluwer; 2018:309–334, 353–362.
2. AIUM practice parameter for the performance of diagnostic and screening ultrasound examinations of the abdominal aorta in adults. https://www.aium.org/resources/guidelines/abdominalAorta.pdf. Accessed September 15, 2018.
3. Penny SM. *Examination Review for Ultrasound: Abdomen & Obstetrics and Gynecology*. 2nd ed. Philadelphia, PA: Wolters Kluwer; 2018:151–167.
4. Rumack CM, Wilson SR, Charboneau JW, Levine D. *Diagnostic Ultrasound*. 4th ed. Philadelphia, PA: Elsevier; 2011:447–485.
5. Sanders RC, Hall-Terracciano B. *Clinical Sonography: A Practical Guide*. 5th ed. Philadelphia, PA: Wolters Kluwer; 2016:381–389, 488–494, 536–538.

7. Abdominal Aorta

CHAPTER 8

Gastrointestinal Tract

INTRODUCTION

Though sonography is somewhat limited in its capacity for the analysis of the gastrointestinal (GI) tract, there are several examinations in which sonography excels. For example, pyloric stenosis, intussusception, and appendicitis are three diagnoses that can be achieved solely with sonography. This chapter will include these three frequently conducted examinations and more information vital for the abdominal sonographer to appreciate in regards to sonography of the GI tract.

AIUM RECOMMENDATION FOR SONOGRAPHY OF THE GI TRACT[1]

- Assess the GI tract in the following manner:
  - When there is concern for bowel pathology, the bowel may be evaluated for wall thickening, dilatation, muscular hypertrophy, masses, vascularity, and other abnormalities.
  - Sonography of the pylorus and surrounding structures may be indicated in the evaluation of the vomiting infant.
  - Graded compression sonography aids in the visualization of the appendix and other bowel loops.
  - Measurements may aid in determining bowel wall thickening, and color or power Doppler imaging may be helpful in assessing hypervascularity.

ESSENTIAL ANATOMY AND PHYSIOLOGY OF THE GI TRACT[2-4]

- General bowel anatomy and physiology
  - The major sections of the GI tract include the mouth, esophagus, stomach, small intestine, and the large intestine or colon (Fig. 8-1).

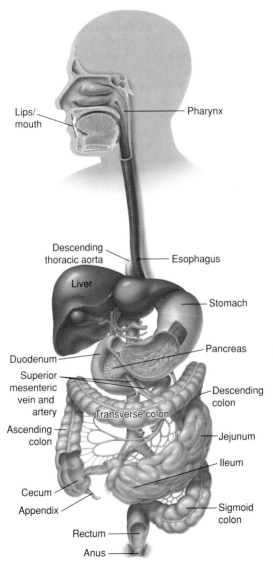

Figure 8-1. Gastrointestinal tract anatomy. (Reprinted with permission from Kawamura D, Nolan T, eds. *Abdomen and Superficial Structures*. 4th ed. Philadelphia, PA: Wolters Kluwer; 2017.)

- The movement of foods and waste products through the GI tract is via segmentation, contractile motion, and peristalsis.
- The stomach provides a temporary storage place for ingested foods and liquids.
- The majority of digestion and nutrient absorption occurs in the small intestines.
- The small intestine can be divided into the duodenum, jejunum, and ileum.
- The colon, which provides a frame around the small intestine, is responsible for water absorption and the creation of feces.
- The colon can be divided into the cecum, ascending colon, transverse colon, descending colon, rectum, and anus.
- The layers of the bowel wall include the superficial mucosa, deep mucosa, submucosa, muscularis propria, and serosa. These layers typically offer what is referred to as gut signature with sonography **(Figs. 8-2 and 8-3)**.

- Anatomy and physiology of infantile hypertrophic pyloric stenosis (IHPS)[2,3,5]
  - The stomach consists of the fundus, body, and pyloric region or pylorus; the latter is the most distal portion **(Fig. 8-4)**.
  - The pylorus consists of the pyloric antrum, which is the opening to the body of the stomach, and the pyloric canal, which is the pathway to the duodenum.
  - The pyloric sphincter is typically located slightly right lateral of the midline of the abdomen, and it controls gastric emptying and is located between the pylorus and the proximal portion of the duodenum.
  - IHPS is a defect in the contractility of the pyloric sphincter of the stomach whereby the sphincter does not permit proper gastric emptying, thus resulting in a gastric outlet obstruction **(Fig. 8-5)**.
  - IHPS can lead to projectile vomiting, severe dehydration, and weight loss.

- Anatomy and physiology of intussusception
  - Intussusception is the invagination or telescoping of a proximal section of bowel into a distal section.

Gastrointestinal wall

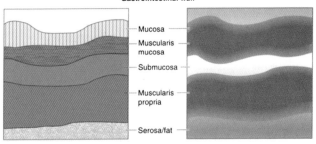

Figure 8-2. Intestinal wall layers. Diagram showing the components of the intestinal wall with the associated sonographic appearance. (Reprinted with permission from Sanders RC, ed. *Clinical Sonography: A Practical Guide.* 5th ed. Philadelphia, PA: Wolters Kluwer; 2015.)

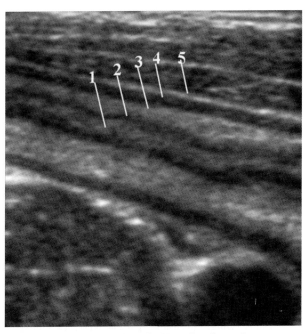

Figure 8-3. Gut signature. Stratified bowel wall, gut signature. 1: Echogenic superficial mucosa. 2: Hypoechoic deep (muscularis) mucosa. 3: Echogenic submucosa. 4: Hypoechoic muscularis propria. 5: Echogenic serosa. (Image courtesy of Kassa Darge, MD.)

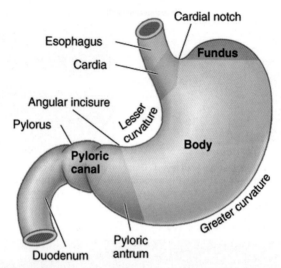

Figure 8-4. Anatomy of the stomach. (Reprinted with permission from Moore KL, Agur AM, Dalley AF, eds. *Essential Clinical Anatomy*. 5th ed. Philadelphia, PA: Wolters Kluwer Health/Lippincott Williams & Wilkins; 2014.)

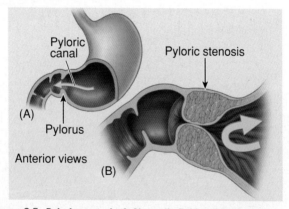

Figure 8-5. Pyloric stenosis. A: Normally fluid and food products are allowed to travel freely through the pyloric canal (*arrow*). **B:** With pyloric stenosis, the pyloric sphincter muscles are thickened and produce a gastric outlet obstruction, inhibiting the fluid and food products from exiting the stomach. (Reprinted with permission from Moore KL, Dalley AF, Agur AM, eds. *Clinically Oriented Anatomy*. 7th ed. Philadelphia, PA: Wolters Kluwer Health/Lippincott Williams & Wilkins; 2013.)

- The proximal portion of the bowel is referred to as the intussusceptum and the distal portion of the bowel is the intussuscipiens **(Fig. 8-6)**.
- Intussusception can occur at any location, but it most often occurs in the right lower quadrant in the area of the ileocecal valve, and is thus referred to as an ileocolic intussusception.
- Intussusception results in a bowel obstruction and can lead to bowel ischemia and gangrene of the bowel.
- Anatomy and physiology of the appendix[3,6]
  - The appendix is a tubular structure that has a base that opens into the cecum and a head or tip.
  - The appendix is most likely located near the ileocecal valve in the right lower quadrant of the abdomen at an area referred to as McBurney point, but its location can vary.
  - McBurney point is established by drawing an imaginary line from the right anterior superior iliac spine along the spinoumbilical line, with the appendix most likely located one-third of the total distance of the line from the iliac spine **(Fig. 8-7)**.
  - The location of the appendix can vary during pregnancy **(Fig. 8-8)**.
  - The function of the appendix is uncertain, though it may serve as a reservoir for beneficial gut flora, and thus may play a role in gut immunity.

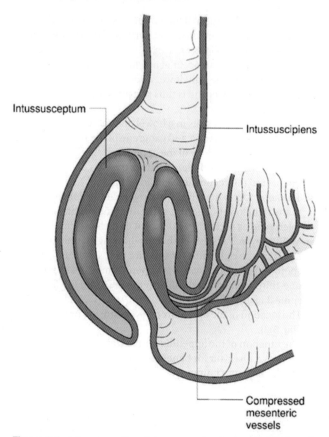

Figure 8-6. **Intussusception. Intussusception is the telescoping of a proximal section of bowel (intussusceptum) into a distal segment (intussuscipiens).** (Reprinted with permission from Fiser SM, ed. *ABSITE Review.* 3rd ed. Philadelphia, PA: Wolters Kluwer Health/Lippincott Williams & Wilkins; 2010.)

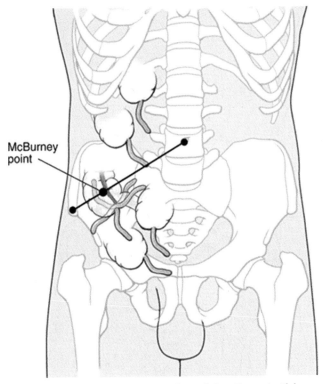

Figure 8-7. Location of McBurney point and the other potential locations of the appendix. McBurney point is established by drawing an imaginary line from the right anterior superior iliac spine along the spinoumbilical line, with the appendix most likely located one-third of the distance from the right iliac spine. (Reprinted with permission from Romans L, ed. *Computed Tomography for Technologists*. Philadelphia, PA: Wolters Kluwer Health/Lippincott Williams & Wilkins; 2010.)

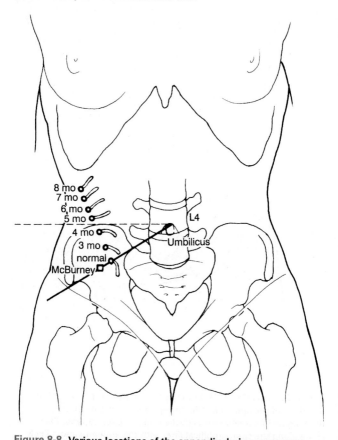

Figure 8-8. Various locations of the appendix during pregnancy.
(Reprinted with permission from Beall M, Ross MH, eds. *Lippincott's Obstetrics Case-Based Review.* Philadelphia, PA: Wolters Kluwer Health/ Lippincott Williams & Wilkins; 2011.)

PATIENT PREPARATION FOR SONOGRAPHY OF THE GI TRACT[3]

- General bowel assessment
  - Sonography should be performed before any imaging requiring barium contrast agents.
  - No preparation is typically required, though if the stomach or duodenum is of interest 10–40 oz of water may be ingested through a straw. Waiting 10–15 min after the administration of the water is suggested before commencing the sonographic assessment of the stomach.*
  - A sonogram of the distal colon could possibly require a water enema, especially if an intraluminal mass is suspected.
- IHPS
  - The infant will need a partially distended stomach.
  - If there is not enough fluid within the pyloric antrum to highlight the pyloric sphincter, then a small amount of glucose solution may be administered orally or via a nasogastric tube.
  - An assistant may be required to hold the infant in the right lateral decubitus position and is most helpful.
- Intussusception
  - No patient preparation is required.
  - Sonography should be performed before any imaging requiring barium contrast agents.
- Appendix
  - No patient preparation is required.
  - Sonography should be performed before any imaging requiring barium contrast agents.

SUGGESTED EQUIPMENT[3,7]

- General bowel assessment
  - Stomach = 3.5- or 5-MHz curved transducer (wall analysis requires higher frequency)
  - Small bowel = 2- to 5-MHz curved transducer or 7.5- to 14-MHz linear transducer
  - Colon = 2- to 5-MHz curved transducer
  - Rectal = 7.5-MHz rectal transducer

---

*Fluid ingestion may be contraindicated in the setting of some clinical situations.

- IHPS
  - 7.5-MHz or higher linear transducer
  - Glucose solution
  - Bottle with nipple
- Intussusception
  - 3.5- or 5-MHz curved transducer
  - 7.5-MHz transducer or higher
- Appendix
  - 7.5-MHz transducer or higher
  - 3.5- or 5-MHz curved transducer

CLINICAL INVESTIGATION FOR SONOGRAPHY OF THE GI TRACT

- Laboratory values are listed in **Table 8.1**.
- Evaluate prior imaging reports and images including CT, MRI, radiography, and any other appropriate tests.
- Critical clinical history questions related to the GI tract
  - General bowel assessment
    - Localized abdominal pain? *General abdominal discomfort may not yield a significant imaging finding. Thus, an inquiry should be made as to the focal point of most pain in the abdomen. Scanning over the area of pain can be constructive.*
    - History of vomiting or diarrhea? *If the patient has a recent history of vomiting, an inquiry of the frequency should be obtained. The incidence of diarrhea should be obtained as well. Inquire about the time in which these disorders began.*
    - Previous abdominal surgery? *This is a vital question for any abdominal imaging study. This also reveals the overall health of the individual.*

Table 8-1	LAB FINDING AND POTENTIAL GI TRACT PATHOLOGY
LAB FINDING	POTENTIAL GI TRACT PATHOLOGY
↑ WBC	Bowel inflammation or infection (e.g., diverticulitis, appendicitis, intussusception, enterocolitis, etc.)

- Unexplained weight loss? *This question can offer a general assessment of the patient's health and could be an indicator for the presence of a possible malignant process.*
- IHPS
  - First-born male? *IHPS most often manifests in first-born, white male babies between 2 and 6 wks following delivery.*
  - Nonbilious, projectile vomiting? *IHPS is most often associated with nonbilious (does not contain bile), projective vomiting.*
  - Weight loss? *Weight loss is often associated with IHPS. Weight gain may be associated with another diagnosis.*
  - Dehydration? *Dehydration is common in infants with IHPS because of the lack of fluid absorption.*
  - Physician prescribed adjustments to feeding (e.g., change in milk formula)? *The infant's pediatrician may initially try to change the infant's milk formula if the child is formula fed.*
  - Physician prescribed acid reflux–reducing medicine? *The infant's pediatrician may initially try to prescribe an acid reflux–reducing medication.*
  - Palpable hypertrophic pyloric muscle? *This is referred to as the olive sign.*
- Intussusception
  - Focal abdominal pain? *If the child can point with one finger to the area that pains him or her the most this is most helpful. Remember, most intussusceptions occur within the right lower quadrant.*
  - Intermittent abdominal pain? *Waves of focal pain in the area of the intussusception may occur.*
  - Red currant jelly stools? *A key clinical feature of intussusception is the presence of red currant jelly stools.*
- Appendix
  - Nausea and vomiting? *With appendicitis, abdominal pain will typically occur before the onset of nausea and vomiting.*

- General abdominal pain? *Appendicitis may initially begin with generalized abdominal pain and then shift to the right lower quadrant.*
- Localized abdominal pain? *An inquiry should be made as to the most focal point of pain in the abdomen. Scanning over the area of pain can be constructive.*
- Rebound tenderness? *Rebound tenderness is pain that is encountered after the removal of pressure.*

NORMAL SONOGRAPHIC DESCRIPTION OF BOWEL[3,4]

- General bowel assessment
  - Normal bowel should be thin walled (Fig. 8-9).
  - Normal bowel is compressible.
  - Normal small bowel is often seen even when not distended with fluid or air (Fig. 8-10).
  - Colon may be seen to contain fluid or air (Fig. 8-11).
  - Peristalsis should be noted.
- IHPS
  - The pyloric muscle should be thin.
  - Upon real-time investigation, the normal pyloric sphincter should be seen opening, allowing fluid to freely pass from the stomach into the duodenum (Fig. 8-12).
- Intussusception
  - Normal bowel should be thin walled and compressible.
  - Peristalsis should be noted.
- Appendix
  - Though the location may vary, the normal appendix may be seen as a blind-ended tube that extends from the base of the cecum in the right lower quadrant (Fig. 8-13).
  - A normal appendix may not be visualized in adults.

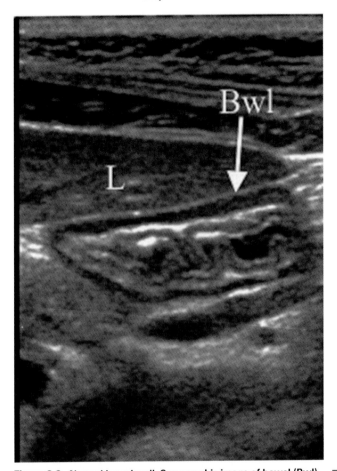

Figure 8-9. **Normal bowel wall. Sonographic image of bowel (Bwl) in the right upper quadrant adjacent to the liver demonstrating the normal sonographic appearance of the echogenicity of the intestinal wall layers.** (Reprinted with permission from Sanders RC, ed. *Clinical Sonography: A Practical Guide.* 5th ed. Philadelphia, PA: Wolters Kluwer; 2015.)

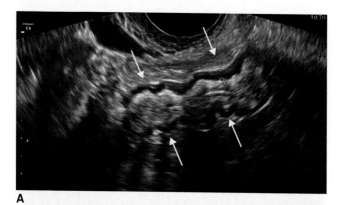

A

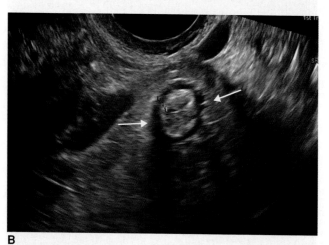

B

Figure 8-10. **Normal small bowel appearance. A:** Longitudinal image of normal small bowel (between *arrows*). **B:** Transverse image of normal small bowel (between *arrows*). The bowel wall is being measured between the *calipers*. (Images courtesy of Barbara Hall-Terracciano.)

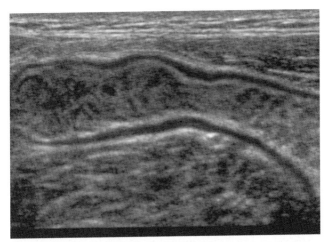

A

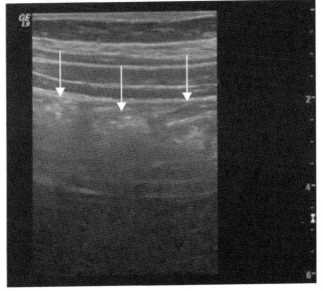

B

Figure 8-11. Normal colon appearance. A, B, C are all representative images of the colon (*arrows*). (Images courtesy of Philips Healthcare, Bothell, WA.) *(continued)*

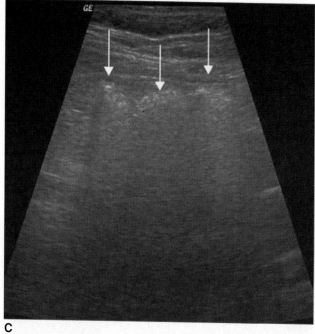

C

Figure 8-11 *(continued).*

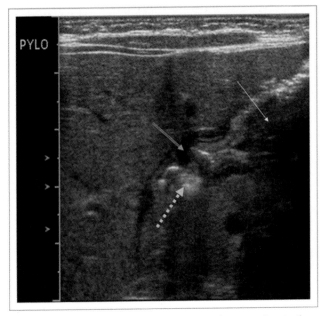

Figure 8-12. Normal pylorus. The *double-lined arrow* points to the normal pylorus, the *thin white arrow* corresponds to fluid within the lumen of the stomach, and the *dotted arrow* points to air entering the first part of the duodenum from the stomach during normal peristalsis. (Image courtesy of Rajesh Krishnamurthy, Radiologist, Texas Children's Hospital, Houston, TX.)

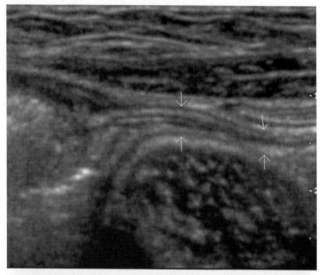

Figure 8-13. Normal appendix. Longitudinal image demonstrates the normal thin-walled appendix (between *arrows*). (Image courtesy of Philips Healthcare, Bothell, WA.)

SUGGESTED PROTOCOL FOR SONOGRAPHY OF THE GI TRACT

- General bowel assessment
  - Survey the area of most discomfort first
    - When a patient is complaining of localized pain, have him or her point to the area of most discomfort and begin your assessment at that point, labeling your image "area of pain."
  - Longitudinal and transverse images
    - Perform an assessment of the bowel in all four quadrants.
    - Utilize graded compression sonography, obtaining pictures in both longitudinal and transverse scan planes with and without compression.
      - Abnormal bowel is typically not compressible and may not yield visual evidence of normal peristalsis.
      - Label your images "with compression" and "without compression."

- Evaluate for altered echogenicity of the bowel wall. A focal area of decreased echogenicity and thickening of the wall is indicative of inflammation.
- Use color Doppler to assess for signs of increased vascularity or hyperemia, which is a sign of inflammation or infection.
- Additional images
  - Several cine loops with and without compression can be beneficial as well.
- IHPS
  - Survey the upper abdomen in transverse and longitudinal
    - Place the infant in the supine position initially.
    - Perform a general survey of the infant's abdomen to assess the distention of the stomach. If the stomach is too distended, distortion of the anatomy can result and could inhibit the visualization of the pyloric region of the stomach.
      - A minimum examination time of 15 min is suggested.[7]
  - Longitudinal pylorus (right lateral decubitus)
    - Place the patient in the right lateral decubitus position. An assistant may be required because the infant will need to remain in this position.
    - While the patient drinks the glucose solution, scan the abdomen actively and assess the pyloric sphincter in real time.
      - A transverse transducer position on the abdomen will provide a longitudinal view of the pylorus (**Fig. 8-14**).
      - The fluid will fill the pyloric region of the stomach and provide an enhanced view of the pyloric sphincter.
      - Fluid seen traveling from the pyloric region of the stomach, through the pyloric canal and pyloric sphincter, and into the duodenum is indicative of a negative study for pyloric stenosis.
      - An enlarged pyloric sphincter will yield the cervix sign in the longitudinal view (Fig. 8-14B).
    - Measure the thickness of the pyloric wall and the length of the pyloric channel (**Fig. 8-15**).
  - Transverse pylorus (right lateral decubitus)
    - A longitudinal transducer position on the abdomen will provide a transverse view of the pylorus (**Fig. 8-16**).

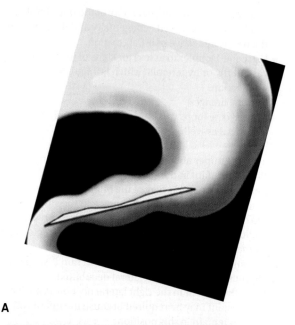

A

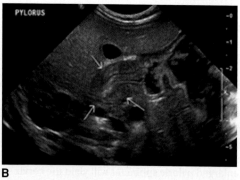

B

Figure 8-14. **Longitudinal pyloric stenosis. A: Longitudinal view of the pylorus is accomplished with a transverse abdominal image. B: Longitudinal sonogram of an enlarged pyloric sphincter (between** *arrows*). (Image A reprinted with permission from Siegel MJ, ed. *Pediatric Sonography.* 4th ed. Philadelphia, PA: Wolters Kluwer Health/Lippincott Williams & Wilkins; 2010; image B reprinted with permission from Penny SM, ed. *Examination Review for Ultrasound.* Philadelphia, PA: Wolters Kluwer Health/Lippincott Williams & Wilkins; 2010.)

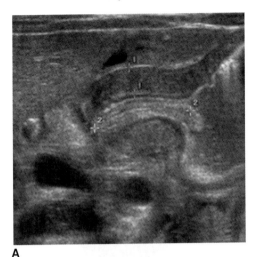

A

B

Figure 8-15. Pyloric stenosis measurements. A: A positive pyloric stenosis will yield a thickened wall that measures ≥3 mm (between **#1** *calipers*) and a channel that measures longer than 17 mm (between **#2** *calipers*). **B:** Since the channel may be curved, a trace method (between *calipers*) may also be used to obtain the length measurement. GB, gallbladder; STOM, stomach; PANC, pancreas.
(Image A reprinted with permission from Siegel MJ, ed. *Pediatric Sonography.* 4th ed. Philadelphia, PA: Wolters Kluwer Health/Lippincott Williams & Wilkins; 2010; image B reprinted with permission from Penny SM, ed. *Introduction to Sonography and Patient Care.* Philadelphia, PA: Wolters Kluwer Health/ Lippincott Williams & Wilkins; 2015.)

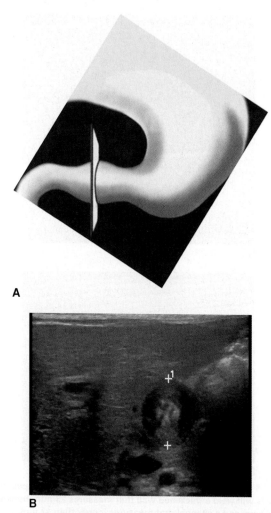

A

B

Figure 8-16. Transverse pyloric stenosis. A: Transverse view of the pylorus is accomplished with a longitudinal abdominal image. B: Transverse sonogram of an enlarged pyloric sphincter (between *plus signs*). (Image A reprinted with permission from Siegel MJ, ed. *Pediatric Sonography*. 4th ed. Philadelphia, PA: Wolters Kluwer Health/ Lippincott Williams & Wilkins; 2010; image B reprinted with permission from Penny SM, ed. *Introduction to Sonography and Patient Care*. Philadelphia, PA: Wolters Kluwer Health; 2015.)

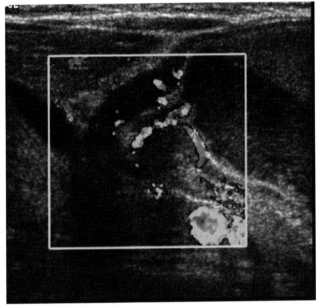

Figure 8-17. Hyperemia with pyloric stenosis. Long-axis color Doppler sonogram shows increased vascularity of the thickened pyloric muscle and underlying submucosa. (Reprinted with permission from Siegel MJ, ed. *Pediatric Sonography*. 5th ed. Philadelphia, PA: Wolters Kluwer; 2018.)

- An enlarged pyloric sphincter will yield the donut sign (Fig. 8-16B).
- Additional images
  - A short cine loop of the fluid moving from the stomach through the pyloric sphincter and into the duodenum can be most beneficial for establishing a definitive diagnosis.
  - Color Doppler can be employed and may yield hyperemia within the enlarged sphincter muscle (Fig. 8-17).
- Intussusception
  - Survey the abdomen in longitudinal and transverse
    - Place the patient in the supine position.

- When a patient is complaining of localized pain, have him or her point to the area of most discomfort and begin your assessment at that point, labeling your image "area of pain."
- Longitudinal and transverse images
  - Utilize the graded compression technique in both longitudinal and transverse scan planes and scan the entire abdomen, keeping in mind that the majority of intussusceptions occur in the right lower quadrant in the area of the ileocecal valve.
  - Label your images "with compression" and "without compression."
    - A positive intussusception will be noncompressible and appear as a doughnut or cinnamon bun in the transverse plane and have a reniform shape in the longitudinal plane (Fig. 8-18).
  - Once identified, measure the intussusception in two orthogonal planes.
  - Utilize color Doppler to assess for evidence of compromised vascular supply or signs of inflammation, the latter of which will increase Doppler signals, which is verification of hyperemia (Fig. 8-19).
- Additional images
  - A short cine loop of the area of interest with and without compression can be beneficial.
- Appendix
  - Survey the abdomen in longitudinal and transverse
    - Place the patient in the supine position.
    - When a patient is complaining of localized pain, have him or her point to the area of most discomfort and begin your assessment at that point, labeling your image "area of pain."
      - Several cine loops with and without compression can be beneficial as well.
  - Longitudinal and transverse images
    - Utilize the graded compression technique in both longitudinal and transverse scan planes and scan the region of interest, keeping in mind that the appendix is typically located within the right lower quadrant.
    - Label your images "with compression" and "without compression."

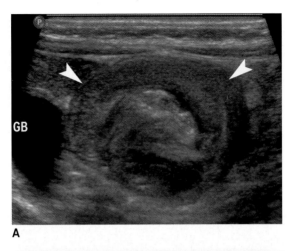

A

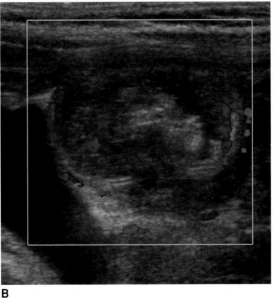

B

Figure 8-18. **Intussusception. A:** The gray scale transverse image of the right upper quadrant shows a large donut-shaped structure (*arrowheads*) with concentric hypoechoic and hyperechoic rings. **B:** The flow seen on a color Doppler transverse image suggests viable bowel. *(continued)*

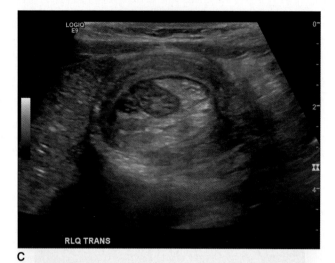

C

D

Figure 8-18 *(continued)*. **C, D: Transverse and longitudinal images from a different patient demonstrating the donut sign in transverse plane and telescoping bowel in longitudinal plane typical of intussusception.** (A and B: Images courtesy of Rechelle Nguyen, Columbus, OH; C and D: Reprinted with permission from Siegel MJ, ed. *Pediatric Sonography*. 5th ed. Philadelphia, PA: Wolters Kluwer Health; 2018.)

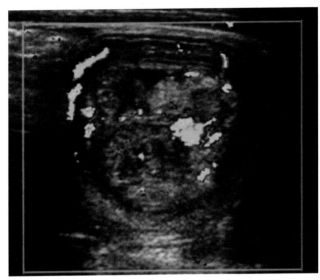

Figure 8-19. Color Doppler of intussusception. Color Doppler sonogram shows flow in the intussuscepted loop of bowel.
(Reprinted with permission from Siegel MJ, ed. *Pediatric Sonography.* 4th ed. Philadelphia, PA: Wolters Kluwer Health/Lippincott Williams & Wilkins; 2010.)

- Identify the ascending colon and slowly manipulate the transducer throughout the right lower quadrant from superior to inferior.
- Measure the appendix when identified.
  - An enlarged appendix will appear as a noncompressible sausage-shaped, blind-ended aperistaltic tube that measures more than 6 mm in diameter (**Figs. 8-20 and 8-21**).
  - An appendicolith may be identified within the abnormal appendix (Fig. 8-20E). An appendicolith is an obstructive stone that often produces shadowing.
  - Patients often complain of rebound tenderness.
- Use color Doppler to assess for the possibility of hyperemia within and/or around the appendix (Fig. 8-20F).

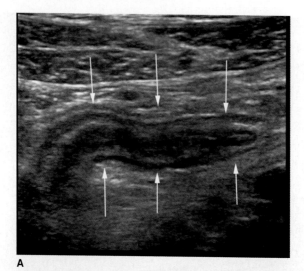

A

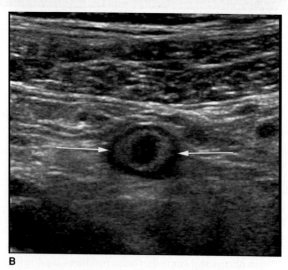

B

Figure 8-20. **Appendicitis. Longitudinal (A) and transverse (B) images of the appendix demonstrate thickening of the wall (*arrows*) consistent with appendicitis.**

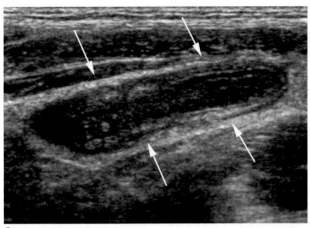

C

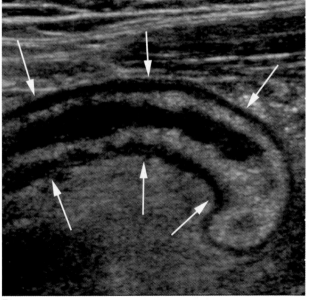

D

Figure 8-20 *(continued).* **C and D: Longitudinal images of two different patients with a dilated, inflamed appendix (between** *arrows***), with a thickened wall and dilatation of the appendiceal lumen.** *(continued)*

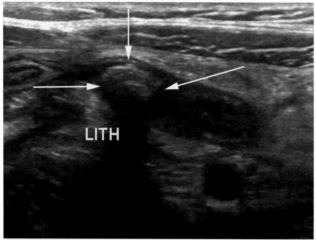

E

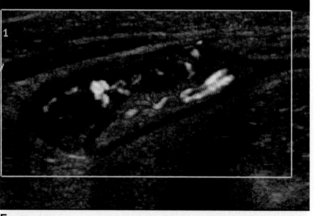

F

Figure 8-20 *(continued).* **E: Longitudinal image of an inflamed appendix containing an echogenic appendicolith (*arrows*). F: Longitudinal image demonstrates hyperemia within an inflamed appendix consistent with appendicitis.** (A–D and F: Images courtesy of Philips Healthcare, Bothell, WA; E: Reprinted with permission from Kawamura D, Nolan T, eds. *Abdomen and Superficial Structures*. 4th ed. Philadelphia, PA: Wolters Kluwer Health; 2017.)

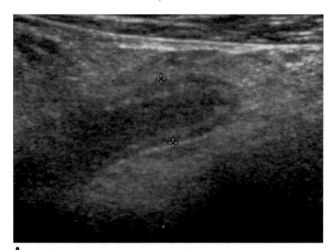

A

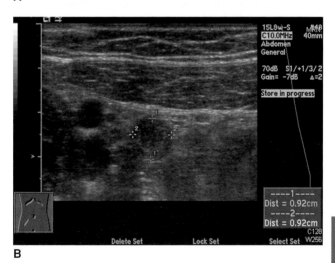

B

Figure 8-21. A: Enlarged abnormal noncompressible appendix (between *calipers*). B: Short axis view of an abnormal appendix (between *calipers*). (Image A reprinted with permission from Britt LD, Peitzman A, Barie P, Jurkovich G, eds. *Acute Care Surgery*. Philadelphia, PA: Wolters Kluwer Health/Lippincott Williams & Wilkins; 2012.)

SCANNING TIPS

- General bowel assessment[8]
  - A lower-frequency transducer may be required in patients with a large body habitus.
  - Minimal peristalsis may exist in the rectum, so manual external pressure applied to the pelvis may assist in the imaging of this area.
- IHPS
  - A good landmark to attempt to identify the pyloric sphincter is the area of the transverse gallbladder. Typically, in the transverse plane to the abdomen, the pyloric region and duodenum are located medial to the gallbladder and anterior to the pancreatic head.
  - Overdistention of the stomach may cause the pyloric sphincter to curl underneath the stomach, thus inhibiting effective visualization and accurate measuring.
  - If the infant becomes restless, an assistant should try to pacify the infant.
- Intussusception
  - An intussusception may appear as a cinnamon bun in the abdomen in the axial plane and have a reniform shape in the longitudinal plane.
- Appendix
  - Posterior manual compression with the nonscanning hand combined with graded compression scanning can be helpful. Perform this analysis with the patient placed in the left lateral decubitus position.
  - Transvaginal sonography may be used to obtain a closer investigation of the appendix in females.

MEASUREMENTS OF THE GI TRACT

- General bowel assessment[3,5]
  - Normal duodenal and small bowel wall = between 2 and 3 mm
  - Normal colon wall nondistended = 4-9 mm
  - Normal colon wall distended = 2-4 mm (when the colon is distended beyond 5 cm)
- Normal pyloric muscle[5]
  - Normal pyloric muscle wall thickness ≤3 mm
  - Normal pyloric channel ≤17 mm

- Pyloric stenosis ≥3 mm in wall thickness and >17 mm in pyloric channel length
- Intussusception[5]
  - Intussuscepted bowel diameter ≥3 cm
- Appendix[3]
  - Normal appendix ≤6 mm in diameter
  - Appendicitis ≥6 mm in diameter

ESSENTIAL GI PATHOLOGY[2]

- General GI pathology
  - Crohn disease **(Fig. 8-22)**—chronic autoimmune disease characterized by period of bowel inflammation
    - Clinical findings
      - ○ Diarrhea
      - ○ Abdominal pain
      - ○ Weight loss
      - ○ Rectal bleeding
    - Sonographic findings
      - ○ Bowel wall thickening
      - ○ Focal areas of noncompressible bowel
      - ○ Bowel wall hyperemia
  - Diverticulitis
    - Clinical findings
      - ○ Constipation or diarrhea
      - ○ Nausea and vomiting
      - ○ Fever
      - ○ Left lower quadrant pain or cramping
    - Sonographic findings
      - ○ Inflamed diverticulum, which appears as an echogenic projection of tissue from the bowel that may shadow or produce ring down artifact
      - ○ Hyperemia within the wall of the affected bowel
  - Colitis
    - Clinical findings
      - ○ Bloody or watery diarrhea
      - ○ Fever
      - ○ Abdominal pain
      - ○ Previous antibiotic therapy
    - Sonographic findings
      - ○ Thickened, hypoechoic colon wall
      - ○ Hyperemia within the colon wall

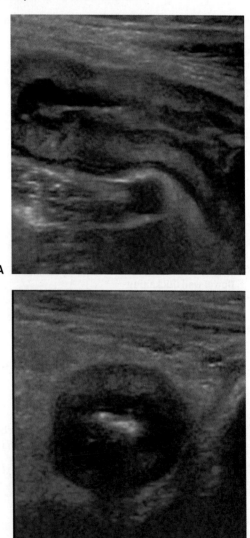

A

B

Figure 8-22. Crohn disease. Longitudinal (A) and transverse (B) images demonstrate hypoechoic thickening of the submucosal layer in the terminal ileum in a patient with Crohn disease.
(Images courtesy of Dr. Taco Geertsma, Hospital Gelderse Vallei, Ede, The Netherlands.)

- Bowel obstruction
  - Clinical findings
    - Abdominal distention
    - Intermittent abdominal pain
    - Constipation
    - Nausea and vomiting
  - Sonographic findings
    - Distended fluid-filled loops of bowel
    - Abrupt termination point of distended bowel
    - Increased peristaltic motion with a to-and-fro motion of intraluminal contents
- IHPS **(Video 8-1)**
  - Clinical findings
    - Nonbilious, projective vomiting
    - First-born, white male patients between the ages of 2 and 6 wks
    - Weight loss
    - Constipation
    - Dehydration
    - Insatiable appetite
    - Palpable olive sign
  - Sonographic findings
    - Target- or doughnut-shaped enlarged pyloric sphincter
    - Cervix appearing enlarged pyloric sphincter
    - Wall of the pylorus measures >3 mm in thickness
    - Length of the pyloric channel measures ≥17 mm
- Intussusception
  - Clinical findings
    - Intermittent, severe abdominal pain
    - Vomiting
    - Palpable abdominal mass
    - Red currant jelly stool
    - Leukocytosis
  - Sonographic findings
    - Noncompressible, target-shaped mass or pseudokidney-shaped mass
    - Altering rings of differing echogenicities (cinnamon bun sign)
    - Intussuscepted bowel diameter will exceed 3 cm

- Appendicitis[2,6] **(Video 8-2)** 🎬
  - Clinical findings
    - ○ Abdominal pain preceded by vomiting
    - ○ General abdominal pain that eventually is restricted to the right lower quadrant
    - ○ Rebound tenderness
    - ○ Possible leukocytosis
    - ○ Fever
  - Sonographic findings
    - ○ Noncompressible, blind-ended tube that measures more than 6 mm from outer wall to outer wall
    - ○ Evidence of an appendicolith
    - ○ Hyperemic flow within the wall of the inflamed appendix
    - ○ Periappendiceal fluid collection
    - ○ Thyroid in the belly sign—hyperechoic edematous connective tissue around the appendix

WHERE ELSE TO LOOK

- IHPS
  - One differential for IHPS is midgut malrotation, which is a rotational abnormality of the small bowel. Midgut malrotation results in bilious vomiting in the first month of life.
    - Midgut malrotation is determined by identifying the relationship between the superior mesenteric artery (SMA) and superior mesenteric vein (SMV). Normally, the SMV is anterior and to the right of the SMA, but with malrotation, this relationship is reversed **(Fig. 8-23)**.[5]
- Appendix
  - Other conditions may mimic appendicitis such as renal stones, pelvic inflammatory disease, and diverticulitis.[9]

IMAGE CORRELATION

- Pyloric stenosis **(Fig. 8-24)**
- Intussusception on radiography and CT **(Fig. 8-25)**
- Appendicitis on CT **(Fig. 8-26)**
- Diverticulitis on CT **(Fig. 8-27)**

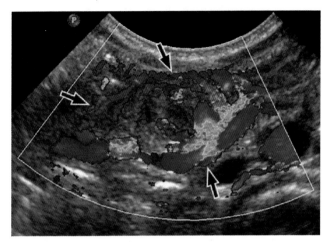

Figure 8-23. Midgut malrotation. Transverse color Doppler ultrasound image shows the whirlpool sign, or swirling of bowel and vessels (*arrows*) around the SMA axis. (Reprinted with permission from Lee E, ed. *Pediatric Radiology: Practical Imaging Evaluation of Infants and Children.* Philadelphia, PA: Wolters Kluwer; 2017.)

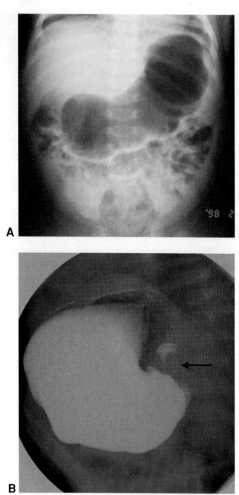

A

B

Figure 8-24. **A: Pyloric stenosis on radiography. B: UGI barium study reveals a pyloric channel that is narrowed and elongated with a double-track appearance (*arrow*) with hypertrophy of the pyloric muscle, consistent with pyloric stenosis.** (Image A reprinted with permission from Fleisher GR, Ludwig S, Baskin MN, eds. *Atlas of Pediatric Emergency Medicine*. Philadelphia, PA: Lippincott Williams & Wilkins; 2004; image B reprinted with permission from Shaffner DH, Nichols DG, eds. *Rogers' Textbook of Pediatric Intensive Care*. 5th ed. Philadelphia, PA: Wolters Kluwer; 2015.)

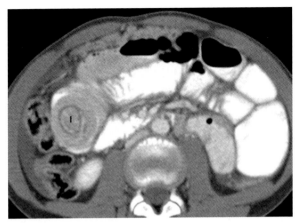

Figure 8-25. Intussusception on CT. Axial contrast-enhanced CT image shows small bowel–small bowel intussusception (I), with normal bowel wall enhancement. (Reprinted with permission from Lee E, ed. *Pediatric Radiology: Practical Imaging Evaluation of Infants and Children.* Philadelphia, PA: Wolters Kluwer; 2017.)

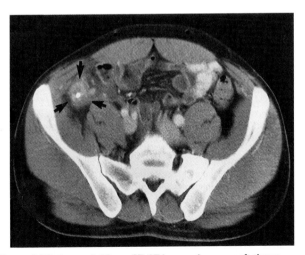

Figure 8-26. Appendicitis on CT. CT image shows a soft tissue inflammatory mass in the right lower quadrant and a calcified fecalith within the thickened appendix (*arrows*). (Reprinted with permission from Daffner RH, Hartman M, eds. *Clinical Radiology.* 4th ed. Philadelphia, PA: Wolters Kluwer Health/Lippincott Williams & Wilkins; 2013.)

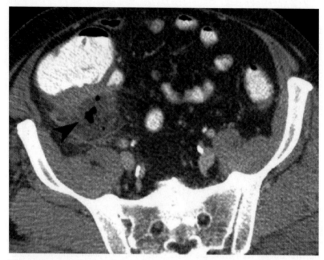

Figure 8-27. Diverticulitis on CT. Diverticulitis with inflamed diverticulum (*arrowhead*). (Reprinted with permission from Singh A, ed. *Gastrointestinal Imaging: The Essentials.* Philadelphia, PA: Wolters Kluwer Health; 2016.)

REFERENCES

1. AIUM practice parameters for the performance of an ultrasound of the abdomen and/or retroperitoneum. http://www.aium.org/resources/guidelines/abdominal.pdf. Accessed June 27, 2018.
2. Penny SM, ed. *Examination Review for Ultrasound: Abdomen & Obstetrics and Gynecology.* 2nd ed. Philadelphia, PA: Wolters Kluwer; 2018:168–178.
3. Kawamura DM, Nolan TD. *Diagnostic Medical Sonography: Abdomen and Superficial Structures.* 4th ed. Philadelphia, PA: Wolters Kluwer; 2018:247–270.
4. Curry RA, Tempkin BB. *Sonography: Introduction to Normal Structure and Function.* 4th ed. St. Louis, MO: Elsevier; 2016:307–330.
5. Seigel MJ. *Pediatric Sonography.* 4th ed. Philadelphia, PA: Wolters Kluwer; 2011:339–383.
6. Penny SM. Imaging the vermiform appendix. *Rad Tech.* 2018;89(6):571–590.
7. Ahuja AT, et al. *Diagnostic and Surgical Imaging Anatomy.* Salt Lake City: Amirsys; 2007:IV140–IV155.
8. Sander RC, Hall-Terracciano BH. *Clinical Sonography: A Practical Guide.* 5th ed. Philadelphia, PA: Wolters Kluwer; 2016:514–524.
9. Federle MP, Jeffrey RB, Woodward PJ. *Diagnostic Imaging: Abdomen.* 2nd ed. Canada: Amirsys; 2010: II-6-26.

CHAPTER 9

Male Pelvis

INTRODUCTION

This chapter provides an overview of the AIUM practice parameters for a sonogram of the scrotum, including a proposed protocol, and the most common pathologies such as epididymitis and testicular torsion. A brief introduction to sonography of the penis is provided as well.

AIUM RECOMMENDATION FOR SONOGRAPHY OF THE SCROTUM[1]

- Assess the scrotum in the following manner:
  - Evaluate the scrotum because of scrotal pain, testicular trauma, ischemia/torsion, and infectious or inflammatory disease.
  - Assess the scrotum for signs of inguinal, intrascrotal, or intratesticular masses.
  - Evaluate the scrotum for signs of hernias and varicoceles.
  - Assess for complications resulting in male infertility and for signs of disorders of sexual development.
  - Examine the scrotum for the localization of nonpalpable testes.
  - Evaluate the scrotum for occult primary tumors associated with metastatic germ cell tumors or retroperitoneal adenopathy.
  - Follow up on patients with sonography for pre-existing scrotal pathology and other abnormalities noted on other imaging studies.

ESSENTIAL ANATOMY AND PHYSIOLOGY OF THE MALE PELVIS[2]

- Anatomy and Physiology of the Male Pelvis
  - Scrotum and Testes:

- The paired testicles initially develop within the upper abdomen and then descend into the scrotum either before birth or shortly thereafter (**Fig. 9-1**). An undescended testicle, a condition referred to as cryptorchidism, is one that is located outside of the scrotum, most likely within the ipsilateral inguinal canal.
- The scrotum is a sack of cutaneous tissue that contains the testicles. The purpose of the scrotum is to attempt to regulate the temperature of the testicles.
- The testicles are normally located within separate compartments by internal and external bands of tissue.
- The testicles function as both endocrine and exocrine glands. The endocrine function is to produce testosterone, while the exocrine function is the production of sperm.
- Spermatogenesis occurs in the seminiferous tubules. These tubules ultimately converse at the rete testis, located within the mediastinum testis.
- The spermatic cord is a structure that travels through the inguinal canal. It contains the testicular veins and arteries, nerves, lymph nodes, and musculature.
- The epididymides are paired structures located adjacent to the testicles that store and transport sperm.
- The epididymis has a head, body, and tail. The head is located more superiorly, while the body travels posteriorly to meet with the tail at the base or the inferior aspect of the testis (see Fig. 9-1).
- There are several testicular appendages, including the appendix testis and the appendix epididymis. These appendages are better visualized when a hydrocele, a fluid collection around the testicle, is present (**Fig. 9-2**).
- Penis:
  - The penis is a primary sex organ.
  - The penis consists of three cylindrical bands of tissue: one corpus spongiosum and two corpus cavernosa (pleural for cavernosum) (**Fig. 9-3**).
  - The corpus spongiosum contains the male urethra and is located ventrally.
  - The corpus cavernosa contain the cavernosal arteries of the penis.

The Testis

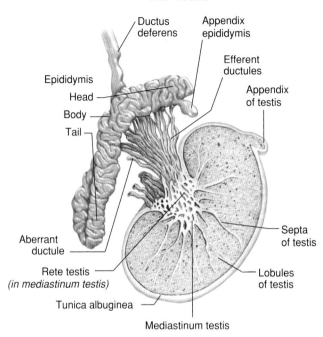

Ductus deferens

Appendix epididymis

Efferent ductules

Appendix of testis

Epididymis

Head

Body

Tail

Aberrant ductule

Rete testis
(in mediastinum testis)

Tunica albuginea

Septa of testis

Lobules of testis

Mediastinum testis

Figure 9-1. Anatomy of the testicle and epididymis. (Reprinted with permission from Anatomical Chart Company. *Understanding Erectile Dysfunction Anatomical Chart.* Philadelphia, PA: Lippincott Williams & Wilkins; 2003.)

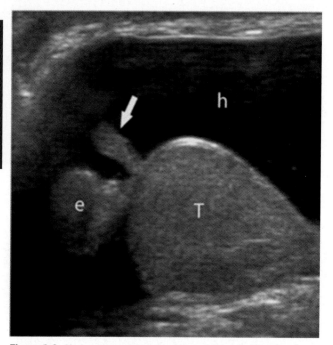

Figure 9-2. Hydrocele and the appendix epididymis. A large hydrocele (h) is noted surrounded this testicle (T). The head of the epididymis (e) and the appendix epididymis (*arrow*) can be seen as well. (Reprinted with permission from Brant WE, Helms C, eds. *Fundamentals of Diagnostic Radiology.* 4th ed. Philadelphia, PA: Wolters Kluwer Health/Lippincott Williams & Wilkins; 2012.)

Cross section of the Penis

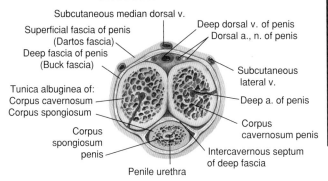

Subcutaneous median dorsal v.

Superficial fascia of penis (Dartos fascia)

Deep fascia of penis (Buck fascia)

Tunica albuginea of:
Corpus cavernosum
Corpus spongiosum

Corpus spongiosum penis

Penile urethra

Deep dorsal v. of penis

Dorsal a., n. of penis

Subcutaneous lateral v.

Deep a. of penis

Corpus cavernosum penis

Intercavernous septum of deep fascia

Figure 9-3. Cross section of the penis. (Reprinted with permission from Anatomical Chart Company. *Male Reproductive System Anatomical Chart.* Philadelphia, PA: Lippincott Williams & Wilkins; 2000.)

- When sexual arousal occurs, the arteries in the penis dilate and restrict venous drainage, ultimately resulting in an erection.

PATIENT PREPARATION FOR SONOGRAPHY OF THE SCROTUM

- No patient preparation is typically required for a sonogram of the male pelvis.

SUGGESTED EQUIPMENT[1]

- 7-MHz or higher linear array transducer for the scrotum and/ or penis
- A curvilinear or vector transducer with lower frequencies may be warranted for improved penetration and a larger field of view, especially in cases of large hydroceles of the scrotum.
- Doppler frequency settings should be optimized (typically between 5 and 10 MHz).
- Towels are often required for patients' positioning (**Fig. 9-4**).
  - Place one towel between the patient's legs, elevating the scrotum and placing it on the towel. This will prospectively demobilize the testicles.
  - Have the patient place his penis on his abdomen, and then drape another towel over the patient's penis in order to

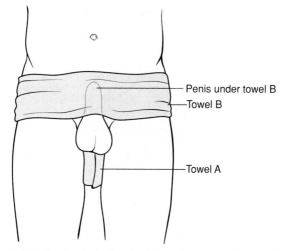

Penis under towel B
Towel B

Towel A

Figure 9-4. Draping technique for a scrotal sonogram. Place one towel between the patient's legs, elevating the scrotum and placing it on the towel. This will prospectively demobilize the testicles. Have the patient place his penis on his abdomen, and then drape another towel over the patient's penis in order to remove it from the field of view, tucking the ends of that towel under the patient's buttocks. The patient could also elevate his scrotum between his legs and cross his ankles in order to stabilize the testes.

remove it from the field of view, tucking the ends of that towel under the patient's buttocks.
- The patient may also assist by holding the towel in place with his hands next to his hips.
- Having the patient cross his legs may help to demobilize the testicles.

CLINICAL INVESTIGATION FOR SONOGRAPHY OF THE MALE PELVIS

- Laboratory values are listed in **Table 9-1:**
- Evaluate prior imaging reports and images including CT, MRI, radiography, and any other appropriate tests.
- Critical clinical history questions related to the scrotum
  - How long have you been hurting? *The extent of time in which pain has occurred is relevant when examining the testicles because a sustained and nagging pain may*

Table 9-1	LAB FINDINGS AND POSSIBLE ASSOCIATED SCROTAL PATHOLOGY
LAB FINDING	POTENTIAL PATHOLOGY
↑ WBC (leukocytosis)	Epididymitis, orchitis, epididymo-orchitis
↑ AFP, hCG, LDH	Used as tumor markers for testicular cancers

9. Male Pelvis

be associated with an ongoing infection, while a sudden extreme onset of pain may be associated with testicular torsion. Unfortunately, the clinical features of these abnormalities can overlap.

- On which side is the pain? *Some sonographers prefer to begin the examination with the asymptomatic testis in order to establish a normal baseline.*
- Where is the pain? *While some patients may claim to have general testicular pain, occasionally testicular pain can be localized for some abnormalities. For example, torsion of the appendix testis often presents with localized pain in the upper pole of the testis.*
- Can you feel the mass and how was it discovered? *It is important to appreciate the initial discovery of the mass. For example, did the patient feel the mass or did his doctor?*
- How long have you had the mass? *This relates to determining if the condition is chronic or acute.*
- Have you had a vasectomy? *The epididymis in patients who have had a vasectomy appears sonographically altered. Most often, the epididymis is often larger in size, may be heterogeneous, and contain small cysts. Within the testes, there may be signs of cysts within the mediastinum testes and granulomas.*

NORMAL SONOGRAPHIC DESCRIPTION OF THE SCROTUM[2,3]

- Testicles and scrotum
  - The normal testes are composed of medium- to low-level echoes, similar to that of the thyroid gland.
  - Often the echogenic configuration of the mediastinum testis can be seen as a linear structure in the longitudinal

plane or a triangular or square-shaped structure in the transverse plane **(Fig. 9-5)**.

- The parenchyma of both testicles should be isoechoic.
- The epididymis may be isoechoic or slightly more echogenic compared to the normal testicle.
- A minimal amount of anechoic fluid may be noted around each testicle.

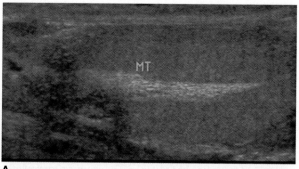

A

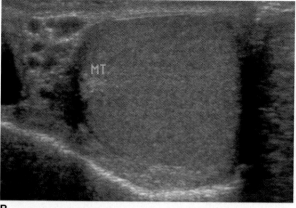

B

Figure 9-5. **Sonographic appearance of the mediastinum testis. A,B: The mediastinum testis (MT) in noted in figure A in the longitudinal plane, while it is demonstrated in figure B in the transverse plane.** (Reprinted with permission from Kawamura D, Lunsford B, eds. *Abdomen and Superficial Structures.* 3rd ed. Philadelphia, PA: Wolters Kluwer Health/Lippincott Williams & Wilkins; 2012.)

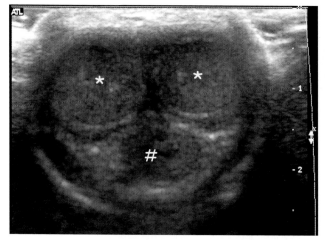

Figure 9-6. Transverse sonographic image of the penis. In this image, the two corpus cavernosa are identified by the *asterisks*, while the spongiosum is indicated by the *hash*. (Reprinted with permission from Penny S, ed. *Examination Review for Ultrasound: Abdomen and Obstetrics and Gynecology.* 2nd ed. Philadelphia, PA: Wolters Kluwer; 2017.)

- Penis
  - The spongiosum is elliptical in shape and consists of medium- to low-level echoes, whereas the paired cavernosa will appear similar to the spongiosum but more oval in shape **(Fig. 9-6)**.

SUGGESTED PROTOCOL FOR SONOGRAPHY OF THE SCROTUM

- The patient is asked to remove his clothing from the waist down and placed in the supine position. Draping instructions are provided in Figure 9-4.
- Scrotum
  - Image each testicle in both the longitudinal and transverse planes **(Fig. 9-7)**. A brief survey can be performed in either plane.
  - Obtain a brief cine loop of the scrotum **(Video 9-1)**.
- Transverse scrotum
  - Obtain an image of both testicles to compare the echogenicity, recalling that the testes should be isoechoic and homogeneous in echotexture **(Fig. 9-8)**.

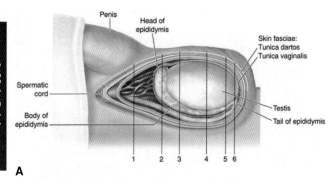

A

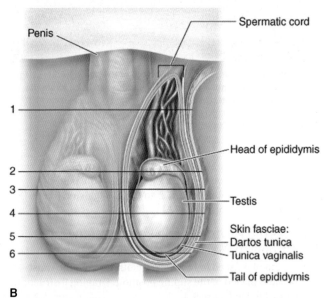

B

Figure 9-7. A: Longitudinal scanning survey for the testes. 1, Spermatic cord; 2, Head of epididymis; 3, Testis—superior; 4, Testis—mid; 5, Testis—inferior; 6, Tail of epididymis. Note that the body of the epididymis is seen in sections 3–5. B: Transverse scanning survey protocol for the testis. 1, Spermatic cord; 2, Head of epididymis; 3, Testis—superior; 4, Testis—mid; 5, Testis—inferior; 6, Tail of epididymis. The body of the epididymis is seen in sections 3–5. (Reprinted with permission from Kawamura D, Nolan T, eds. *Abdomen and Superficial Structures.* 4th ed. Philadelphia, PA: Wolters Kluwer; 2017.)

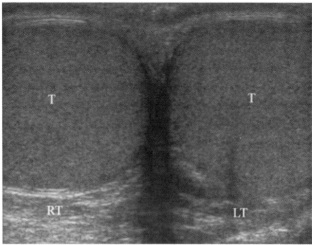

A

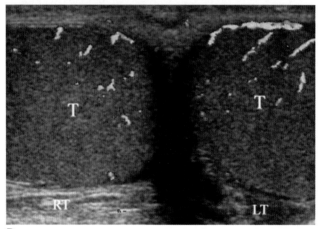

B

Figure 9-8. **Transverse of both testicles with and without color Doppler. A: Transverse image of normal bilateral right (RT) and left (LT) testes (T) demonstrating similar homogeneous echogenicity. B: Transverse image of normal bilateral right (RT) and left (LT) testes (T) demonstrating normal flow bilaterally.** (Reprinted with permission from Kawamura D, Nolan T, eds. *Abdomen and Superficial Structures.* 4th ed. Philadelphia, PA: Wolters Kluwer; 2017.)

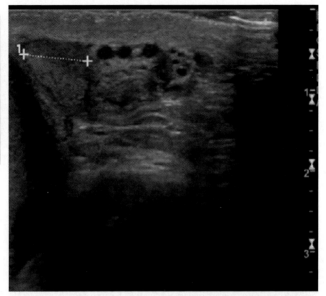

Figure 9-9. Transverse epididymal head with measurement. The epididymal head (between *calipers*) is demonstrated in this image in transverse.

- Transverse scrotum with color Doppler (see Fig. 9-8)
  - After obtaining an image of both testicles, apply color Doppler to both simultaneously to assess for vascular symmetry. While comparatively an absent or noticeable decreased flow may suggest torsion, excessive flow or hyperemia may suggest infection.
- Transverse (right or left) epididymal head (repeat on the contralateral side)
  - Obtain an image of the epididymal head (Fig. 9-9).
  - Measure the epididymal head if requested.
    - Color Doppler may also provide information regarding hyperemia of the epididymis associated with epididymitis.
- Transverse superior (right or left) testicle (repeat on the contralateral side)
  - Scanning from superior to inferior, obtain an image of the superior portion of the testicle.

- Transverse mid (right or left) testicle with and without measurement (repeat on the contralateral side) **(Fig. 9-10)**
  - Obtain an image of the widest dimension of the testicle.
- Transverse mid (right or left) testicle with color Doppler and pulsed-wave Doppler (repeat on the contralateral side) **(Fig. 9-11)**
  - Obtain an image of the color Doppler signals within the testicle.
  - Obtain an image of the arterial, and if requested venous, pulsed-wave Doppler signals within the testicle.
  - Utilize power Doppler if necessary.
- Transverse inferior (right or left) testicle (repeat on the contralateral side)
  - Acquire an image of the inferior portion of the testicle.
  - Scan completely through the testicle.
    - At this time, the tail of the epididymis may be visualized.
  - Obtain a color Doppler image of the tail of the epididymis.

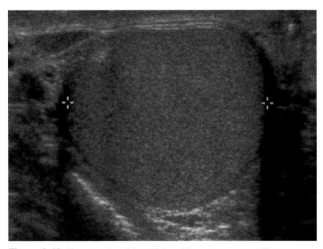

Figure 9-10. Transverse mid testicle with measurement. Transverse measurement of the testis (between *calipers*). (Reprinted with permission from Kawamura D, Lunsford B, eds. *Abdomen and Superficial Structures.* 3rd ed. Philadelphia, PA: Wolters Kluwer Health/Lippincott Williams & Wilkins; 2012.)

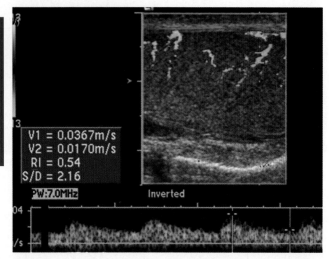

Figure 9-11. Mid testicle with spectral and color Doppler. Normal spectral waveform of intratesticular artery with low-resistance flow. (Reprinted with permission from Kawamura D, Lunsford B, eds. *Abdomen and Superficial Structures.* 3rd ed. Philadelphia, PA: Wolters Kluwer Health/ Lippincott Williams & Wilkins; 2012.)

- Longitudinal (right or left) epididymal head (repeat on the contralateral side) **(Fig. 9-12)**
  - Obtain an image of the epididymal head in longitudinal.
  - Measure the head of epididymis.
  - Obtain a color Doppler image of the epididymal head.
- Longitudinal (right or left) testicle with and without measurements (repeat on the contralateral side) **(Fig. 9-13)**
  - Obtain the longest dimension of the testicle and measure the length and anteroposterior dimensions.
  - Do not include any part of the epididymis in these measurements.
- Longitudinal (right or left) testicle with color Doppler and pulsed-wave Doppler (repeat on the contralateral side)
  - If not obtained in transverse, obtain an image of the color Doppler signals within the testicle.
  - Obtain an image of the arterial, and if requested venous, pulsed-wave Doppler signals within the testicle.
  - Utilize power Doppler if necessary.

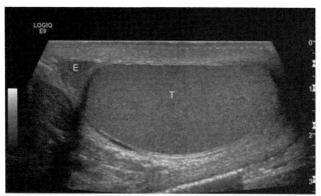

A

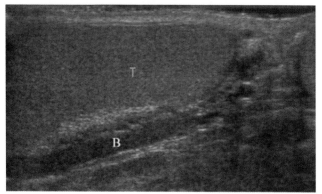

B

Figure 9-12. **Longitudinal epididymus. A: Longitudinal image of normal testis (T) and epididymal head (E). B: Longitudinal image of normal testis (T) with the body of epididymis (B).** *(continued)*

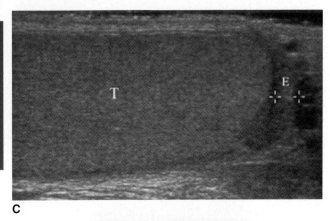

C

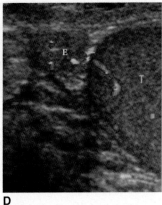

D

Figure 9-12 *(continued).* **C: Longitudinal image of normal testis (T) and tail of epididymis (E). D: Longitudinal color image of testis (T) with normal flow in the epididymis (E).** (Reprinted with permission from Kawamura D, Nolan T, eds. *Abdomen and Superficial Structures.* 4th ed. Philadelphia, PA: Wolters Kluwer; 2017.)

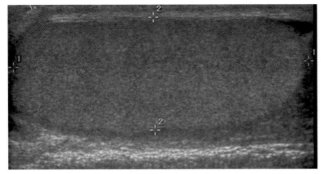

Figure 9-13. Longitudinal testicle with measurement. Longitudinal measurement of the testis (between *calipers*). (Reprinted with permission from Kawamura D, Lunsford B, eds. *Abdomen and Superficial Structures*. 3rd ed. Philadelphia, PA: Wolters Kluwer Health/Lippincott Williams & Wilkins; 2012.)

- Longitudinal (right or left) testicle medial (repeat on the contralateral side)
  - Scan through the testicle medially, obtaining several images.
- Longitudinal (right or left) testicle lateral (repeat on the contralateral side)
  - Scan through the testicle laterally, obtaining several images.
- Additional images:
  - Palpable scrotal masses may be best demonstrated by having the patient point with his finger, or if possible, hold the mass between two of his fingers while you scan.
  - Inguinal canal images can be obtained to analyze and demonstrate the spermatic cord.

SCANNING TIPS[3]

- Extended field of view images may be helpful to demonstrate the entire length of the testicles.
- For comparison purposes, dual images may be utilized to best demonstrate the echogenicity of both testicles.
- When anechoic vascular tubes are noted adjacent to the testicle (varicocele), the patient should perform the Valsalva

maneuver. To do this, have him tighten his abdominal muscles. This will increase intrabdominal pressure. Obtain color Doppler images with and without the Valsalva maneuver.
- Upright scanning may be performed when a varicocele is suspected.
- It is important to assess the thickness of the scrotal wall. Thickening may be indicative of an infectious process.
- Utilize a curved transducer for large hydroceles in order to demonstrate the pathology and identify the testicles.
- Utilize a stand-off device or a large mound of gel to demonstrate superficial abnormalities.

NORMAL MEASUREMENTS OF THE SCROTUM[1–3]

- Adult testicle:
  - 3–5 cm in length
  - 2–4 cm in width
  - 3 cm in thickness
- Epididymal head:
  - 10–12 mm
- Scrotal wall:
  - 2–8 mm in thickness
- Testicular volume:
  - Length × width × height × 0.52 (ellipsoid formula)
  - Length × width × height × 0.71

ESSENTIAL SCROTAL PATHOLOGY[2]

- Testicular torsion—twisting of the testicle on its vascular pedicle that causes compromised vascular supply and venous drainage (Fig. 9-14)
  - Clinical findings:
    - Acute testicular pain often at rest
    - Swollen testis/scrotum
    - Nausea and vomiting
    - Painful testes positioned higher and horizontally
  - Sonographic findings:
    - Enlargement of the spermatic cord, epididymis, and testis
    - Thickened scrotal wall
    - Hypoechoic or heterogeneous testis
    - Reactive hydrocele

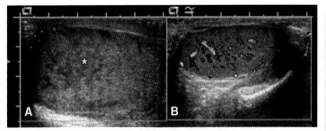

Figure 9-14. Testicular torsion. Longitudinal color Doppler sonogram of the right (A) and left (B) testicles demonstrates right testicular enlargement and heterogeneity (*asterisk*) as well as absent blood flow, consistent with testicular torsion. The left testicle is normal. (Reprinted with permission from Lee E, ed. *Pediatric Radiology: Practical Imaging Evaluation of Infants and Children.* 1st ed. Philadelphia, PA: Wolters Kluwer; 2017.)

- Absent intratesticular flow with color Doppler
- Decreased intratesticular flow with color Doppler compared to the asymptomatic testes
- Epididymitis (epididymo-orchitis)—inflammation of the epididymis and/or testicle **(Fig. 9-15)**
  - Clinical findings:
    - Acute testicular pain
    - Leukocytosis
    - Fever
    - Dysuria
    - Urethral discharge
    - Scrotal wall edema (erythema)
  - Sonographic findings:
    - Enlargement of the affected portion of the epididymis
    - Hypoechoic testis (orchitis)
    - Hyperemia within the epididymis and/or testis
    - Thickened scrotal wall
    - Reactive hydrocele
- Varicocele—dilated veins within the scrotum (most likely on the left) **(Fig. 9-16)**
  - Clinical findings:
    - Often asymptomatic but may cause discomfort
    - Fullness within the scrotum
    - Possible infertility

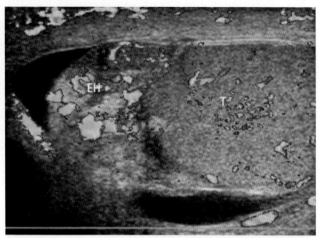

A

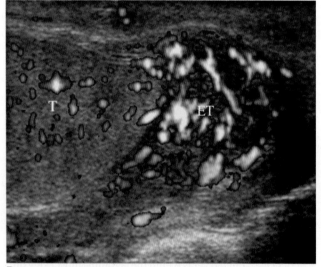

B

Figure 9-15. Epididymitis and orchitis. A: Sagittal color Doppler image of a hyperemic epididymal head (EH). B: Sagittal power Doppler image of a hyperemic epididymal tail (ET).

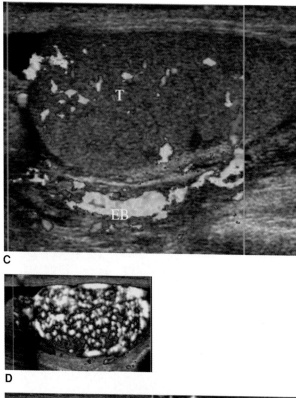

C

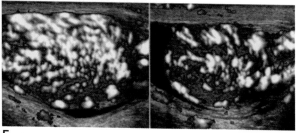

D

E

Figure 9-15 *(continued)*. **C: Sagittal color Doppler image a hyperemic epididymal body (EB). D, E: Power Doppler images of a hyperemic testicle, indicating orchitis.** (Reprinted with permission from Kawamura D, Nolan T, eds. *Abdomen and Superficial Structures*. 4th ed. Philadelphia, PA: Wolters Kluwer; 2017.)

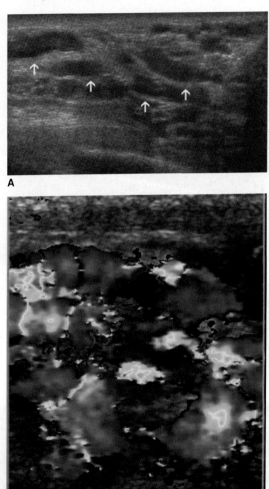

A

B

Figure 9-16. Varicocele. A: Sonographic demonstration of multiple
anechoic tubular structures representing veins within the scrotum
adjacent to the testicle are noted. B: Increased vascular flow is
demonstrated within the dilated veins when color Doppler is applied.
(Reprinted with permission from Kawamura D, Nolan T, eds. *Abdomen and
Superficial Structures*. 4th ed. Philadelphia, PA: Wolters Kluwer; 2017.)

- Sonographic findings:
  - Tubular vascular anechoic structures adjacent to the testis
  - Dilated veins within the scrotum that measure greater than 2 mm
  - Distention of the veins occurs with the Valsalva maneuver
- Seminoma (testicular malignancy)
  - Clinical findings:
    - Painless enlargement of the testis
    - Elevated human chorionic gonadotropin
  - Sonographic findings:
    - Solid hypoechoic or heterogeneous mass within the testicle
- Penile trauma
  - Clinical findings:
    - History of hearing an audible popping sound during intercourse
    - Penile erythema (redness) denoting a subcutaneous bleeding area
  - Sonographic findings:
    - Irregular hypoechoic or hyperechoic defect at the site of penile rupture
    - Notable hematoma in the area of erythema

WHERE ELSE TO LOOK

- It may be prudent to briefly survey the retroperitoneum on the ipsilateral side of a varicocele because varicoceles may be associated with retroperitoneal pathology, especially on the right side.
- Assess the inguinal canal of the ipsilateral side for evidence of an undescended testicle if it is absent from the scrotum. The testicle may also be located within the abdomen or pelvis.
- Be sure to analyze the scrotal wall for signs of thickening.
- In cases of suspected hernia, watch the incarcerated bowel for signs of peristalsis.

IMAGE CORRELATION

- Scrotal mass on CT (**Fig. 9-17**)

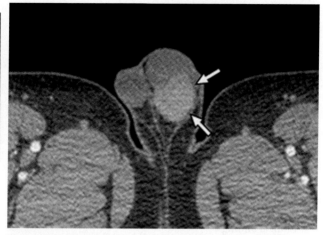

Figure 9-17. **Scrotal mass on CT. Axial contrast-enhanced CT image demonstrates an enhancing left extratesticular scrotal mass (*arrows*).** (Reprinted with permission from Lee E, ed. *Pediatric Radiology: Practical Imaging Evaluation of Infants and Children*. 1st ed. Philadelphia, PA: Wolters Kluwer; 2017.)

REFERENCES

1. AIUM Practice Parameters for the Performance of the Scrotal Ultrasound Examinations. https://www.aium.org/resources/guidelines/scrotal.pdf. Accessed October 18, 2018.
2. Penny SM, ed. *Examination Review for Ultrasound: Abdomen & Obstetrics and Gynecology*. 2nd ed. Philadelphia, PA: Wolters Kluwer; 2018:205–223.
3. Sanders RC, Hall-Terracciano B, eds. *Clinical Sonography: A Practical Guide*. 5th ed. Philadelphia, PA: Wolters Kluwer; 2016:735–746.

CHAPTER 10

Neck and Face

INTRODUCTION

Sonography of the thyroid gland and surrounding area, including an assessment for parathyroid pathology and lymphadenopathy of the neck, is exceedingly common and useful. Sonography can also aid in the guidance of fine-needle aspiration of thyroid lesions. Since sonography can provide a noninvasive analysis of the face, it may be utilized to characterize pathology in this region as well. This chapter will provide protocols for thyroid and parathyroid sonographic analysis, as well as the salivary glands and general neck lymph node locations.

AIUM RECOMMENDATION FOR SONOGRAPHY OF THE NECK AND FACE[1]

- Assess the thyroid and parathyroid in the following manner:
  - Determine the location and characteristics of palpable neck masses.
  - Evaluate for abnormalities identified on another imaging study or assess for evidence of pathology associated with abnormal laboratory findings.
  - Assess the size and location of the thyroid gland.
  - Evaluate the thyroid in patients who have a high risk for thyroid malignancy.
  - Provide follow-up analysis of previously discovered thyroid nodules.
  - Evaluate for signs of recurrent disease or regional nodal metastases.
  - Assess for the location of parathyroid abnormalities in patients with suspected primary or secondary hyperparathyroidism.
  - Assess for the number and size of enlarged parathyroid glands in patients who have undergone previous

parathyroid surgery or ablative therapy with recurrent symptoms of hyperparathyroidism.

- Locate thyroid/parathyroid abnormalities or adjacent cervical lymph nodes for biopsy, ablation, or other interventional procedures.
- Identify unsuspected thyroid pathology after parathyroid localization with a nuclear medicine exam (sestamibi scan) and the localization of autologous parathyroid gland implants.
- Assess the salivary glands in the following manner:
  - Evaluate for enlargement and tenderness of the glands, which may indicate sialadenitis.
  - Assess for signs of abscess formation.
  - Evaluate for swelling and signs of Sjögren disorder.
  - Identify signs of obstructive salivary gland calculus, solitary salivary gland masses or cysts, and oral lesions.

ESSENTIAL ANATOMY AND PHYSIOLOGY OF THE NECK AND FACE[2,3]

- Anatomy and physiology of the thyroid gland
  - The thyroid is located in the anterior neck (**Fig. 10-1**).
  - The thyroid consists of a right and left lobe.
  - The thyroid lobes are connected by a bridge of tissue located anterior to the trachea referred to as the isthmus.
  - Some patients may have a pyramidal lobe, which is a superior extension of the isthmus.
  - The anterior pituitary gland produces thyroid hormone (TSH), which controls the release of hormones by the thyroid.
  - Thyroxine (T_4), triiodothyronine (T_3), and calcitonin are hormones released by the thyroid gland, and they all work together to help regulate metabolism, growth, and development.
  - A surplus of thyroid hormones is referred to as hyperthyroidism and a reduction is referred to as hypothyroidism.
- Anatomy and physiology of the parathyroid glands
  - Most individuals have two pairs of parathyroid glands.
  - The parathyroid glands are often located near the posterior aspect of the midportion of each lobe, and one is often located inferior to each lobe. But there can be some aberrant locations (**Fig. 10-2**).

10. Neck and Face

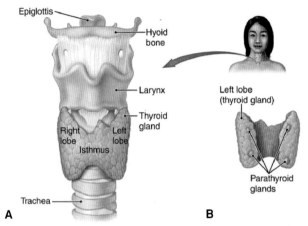

Figure 10-1. Location of the thyroid and common locations for parathyroid glands. A: The thyroid is located anterior to the trachea. B: There are typically two pairs of parathyroid glands. (Reprinted with permission from McConnell TH, Hull KL, eds. *Human Form, Human Function*. 1st ed. Philadelphia, PA: Wolters Kluwer Health/Lippincott Williams & Wilkins; 2011.)

- The parathyroid glands serve the purpose of calcium regulation in the blood.
- An elevation in the serum calcium level is referred to as hypercalcemia, while a reduction in calcium is referred to as hypocalcemia.
- Anatomy and physiology of the lymph nodes of the neck
  - Lymph nodes are important for the functioning of the immune system by acting as filters of foreign materials and abnormal cells.
  - They are small islands of tissue that contain B and T lymphocytes and other white blood cells.
  - Each lymph node consists of an outer cortex and an inner medulla.
  - There exists within the lateral neck a chain of small lymph nodes.
  - The lymph nodes of the neck may be evaluated during a sonogram of the thyroid and may be evaluated sonographically using a numbered region or level method (**Fig. 10-3**).

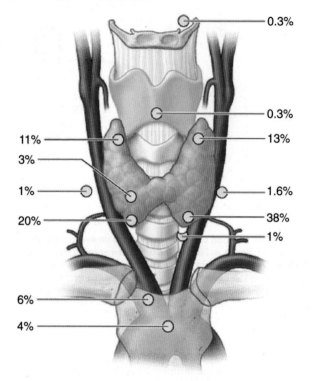

Figure 10-2. Possible locations of the parathyroid glands. (Reprinted with permission from Moore KL, Dalley AF II, Agur AMR, eds. *Clinically Oriented Anatomy.* 8th ed. Philadelphia, PA: Wolters Kluwer; 2017.)

- Anatomy and physiology of the salivary glands
  - The face contains three sets of paired salivary glands: the sublingual glands, the submandibular glands, and the parotid glands (Fig. 10-4).
  - The bilateral parotid glands are the largest of the salivary glands and they are located anterior to the ears on each side of the face.
  - The submandibular glands are located under the mandible bilaterally. They are bordered laterally by the mandibular body and superiorly and medially by the mylohyoid muscle.
  - The sublingual glands are located under the tongue.

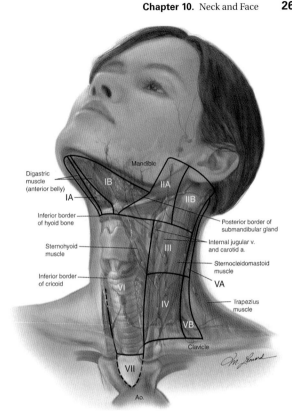

Digastric muscle (anterior belly)

IB

IA

IIA

IIB

Mandible

Inferior border of hyoid bone

Posterior border of submandibular gland

Sternohyoid muscle

Internal jugular v. and carotid a.

III

Inferior border of cricoid

Sternocleidomastoid muscle

VA

VI

IV

VB

Trapezius muscle

Clavicle

VII

Ao.

Figure 10-3. Lymph node regions of the neck. (Reprinted with permission from Myers J, Hanna E, eds. *Cancer of the Head and Neck.* 5th ed. Philadelphia, PA: Wolters Kluwer; 2016.)

10. Neck and Face

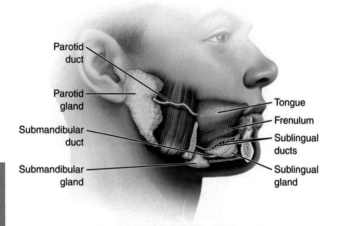

Figure 10-4. Location of the salivary glands. (Reprinted with permission from McConnell TH, Hull KL, eds. *Human Form, Human Function.* 1st ed. Philadelphia, PA: Wolters Kluwer Health/Lippincott Williams & Wilkins; 2011.)

- The primary function of the salivary glands is to produce saliva, which aids in digestion by containing amylase.
- Saliva is transported to the mouth via the salivary ducts.

PATIENT PREPARATION FOR SONOGRAPHY OF THE NECK AND FACE

- No patient preparation is typically required for a sonogram of the neck and face.

SUGGESTED EQUIPMENT[1]

- 8–12 MHz linear transducer.
- Lower frequencies may be warranted in some situations where more penetration is required.
- A stand-off pad or mounded gel is useful for the investigation of superficial pathologies.

CLINICAL INVESTIGATION FOR SONOGRAPHY OF THE NECK AND FACE[2]

- Laboratory values are listed in **Table 10-1.**
- Evaluate prior imaging reports and images including nuclear medicine, CT, MRI, radiography, and any other appropriate tests.

Table 10-1	LAB FINDINGS AND POSSIBLE ASSOCIATED NECK PATHOLOGY

LAB FINDING	POTENTIAL PATHOLOGY
↑ WBC (leukocytosis)	Infection within the neck or face; lymphadenopathy; sialadenitis
↑ Thyroid stimulating hormone (TSH), T_3, T_4	Hyperthyroidism (Graves disease)
↓ Thyroid stimulating hormone (TSH), T_3, T_4	Hypothyroidism (Hashimoto thyroiditis)
↑ Serum calcium	Hyperparathyroidism or parathyroid adenoma
↑ Parathyroid hormone (PTH)	Hyperparathyroidism

- Critical clinical history questions related to the neck and face
  - Thyroid and parathyroid glands
    - Have you had any neck surgeries? *Patients with a history of neck surgeries may have a history of previous thyroid cancer, and thus may only have one lobe or none at all. In this situation, if any exists, residual tissue should be assessed, and the entire neck should be evaluated for possible metastasis to the cervical lymph nodes.*
    - Have you been diagnosed with hyperthyroidism or hypothyroidism? *Both hyperthyroidism and hypothyroidism can alter the sonographic appearance of the thyroid gland.*
    - Do you have a mass in your neck that you can feel? *If so, have the patient indicate the area that is palpable to him or her.*
    - Do you have difficulty breathing or swallowing? *Dyspnea and dysphagia could be caused by an enlarged thyroid gland.*
    - Are you taking any thyroid-related medications? *Levothyroxine sodium (Synthroid) is a commonly prescribed medication used to treat hypothyroidism.*

10. Neck and Face

- Cervical lymph nodes
  - Have you had any neck surgeries? *Patients with a history of neck surgeries may have a history of previous thyroid cancer, and thus may only have one lobe or none at all. In this situation, if any exists, residual tissue should be assessed, and the entire neck should be evaluated for possible metastasis to the cervical lymph nodes.*
  - Do you have a mass in your neck that you can feel? *If so, have the patient indicate the area that is palpable to him or her.*
- Salivary glands
  - Do you have a mass in your face that you can feel? *If so, have the patient indicate the area that is palpable to him or her.*
  - Do you have a history of salivary stones or salivary gland surgery? *Past stones or surgery indicates a history of salivary gland issues. Inquire as to when and what treatment was received for the ailment.*

NORMAL SONOGRAPHIC DESCRIPTION OF THE NECK AND FACE[4]

- Thyroid gland
  - The normal tissue of the thyroid gland is homogeneous and consists of medium- to high-level echogenicities similar to that of the testes **(Fig. 10-5)**.
- Parathyroid glands
  - Normal parathyroid glands are often oval or bean shaped and are isoechoic to the adjacent thyroid tissue.
  - Normal parathyroid glands may not be clearly delineated with sonography.
- Normal cervical lymph nodes
  - Normal cervical lymph nodes tend to measure <1 cm, are oval in shape, hypoechoic, and have an echogenic hilum **(Fig. 10-6)**.
- Salivary glands[4]
  - The normal salivary glands are homogeneous and hyperechoic compared to the adjacent musculature.
  - The parotid gland is round in transverse and elliptical on coronal images.
  - Often, there are several intraparotid lymph nodes **(Fig. 10-7)**.

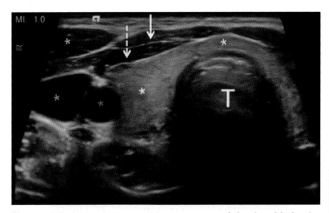

Figure 10-5. Normal sonographic appearance of the thyroid gland.
Transverse sonographic image of the right thyroid lobe (*white asterisk*) demonstrates homogeneous echotexture. The isthmus (*yellow asterisk*) is normal in thickness. Lateral to the thyroid lobe, the common carotid artery (*red asterisk*) and internal jugular vein (*blue asterisk*) are noted. Overlying the gland are strap muscles (*white arrows*), with the sternocleidomastoid muscle (*orange asterisk*) seen more laterally. The trachea (T) is seen in the midline.
(Reprinted with permission from Sanelli P, Schaefer P, Loevner L, eds. *Neuroimaging: The Essentials.* 1st ed. Philadelphia, PA: Wolters Kluwer; 2015.)

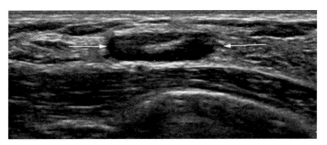

Figure 10-6. Normal lymph node. This image depicts the normal sonographic appearance of a lymph node (between *arrows*). Note the fatty hilum and oval shape. (Image courtesy of Philips Medical Systems, Bothell, WA.)

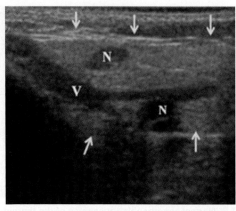

Figure 10-7. Normal parotid gland. Longitudinal scan parallel to the earlobe. In this plane, the gland has an elliptical shape (*arrows*). Note also normal hypoechoic intraparotid lymph nodes (N). The retromandibular vein (V) divides the gland into the superficial lobe anteriorly and deep lobe posteriorly. (Reprinted with permission from Siegel MJ, ed. *Pediatric Sonography.* 4th ed. Philadelphia, PA: Wolters Kluwer Health/Lippincott Williams & Wilkins; 2010.)

SUGGESTED PROTOCOL FOR SONOGRAPHY OF THE NECK AND FACE

- Thyroid gland
  - Survey the thyroid gland
    - Perform the examination with the neck in extension and the patient either supine or semirecumbent.
    - Remove the patient's pillow and place a rolled towel under the patient's neck to assist in neck extension.
    - Survey the thyroid in either the transverse or longitudinal planes.
    - Scan completely through both lobes for a brief assessment of the parenchyma.
    - Scan from superior to inferior in the transverse plane and obtain a short video (**Video 10-1**). 📹
  - Transverse isthmus
    - The thickness (anteroposterior measurement) of the isthmus on the transverse view should be recorded (**Fig. 10-8**).

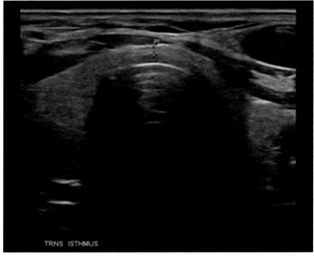

A

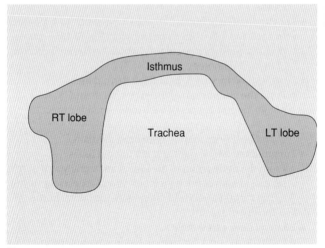

B

Figure 10-8. Transverse thyroid isthmus. A, B: Transverse of the isthmus with anteroposterior thickness measurement (between *calipers*).

- Transverse right and left thyroid lobes
  - Have the patient turn his or her face slightly to the opposite direction that you are examining, if needed.
  - Obtain several images of the superior aspect of each lobe (Fig. 10-9).
  - Obtain an image of the midportion of each lobe with and without a transverse measurement (Fig. 10-10). An anteroposterior measurement can be obtained in the transverse plane as well.
  - Obtain several images of the inferior aspect of each lobe (Fig. 10-11).
- Longitudinal right and left thyroid lobes
  - Lengthening the complete lobe, obtain an image of the midportion of each lobe.
  - Measure the length, and if not obtained in transverse, obtain the anteroposterior dimension of the right lobe (Fig. 10-12).
  - An extended-field-of-view or dual image may be warranted to obtain the full length of enlarged thyroid lobes.
- Longitudinal right and left thyroid lobes with color Doppler
  - Image each lobe with color Doppler (Fig. 10-13).
  - Evaluate for hypervascularity, which can be an indicator of thyroid pathology.
- Longitudinal medial right and left thyroid lobes
  - From the midportion of the lobe scan medially and obtain several images of each lobe's medial aspect (Fig. 10-14).
    ○ Tracheal rings may be visualized medially.
- Longitudinal lateral right and left thyroid lobes
  - From the midportion of the lobe scan laterally and obtain several images of the right lobe's lateral aspect (Fig. 10-15).
    ○ The carotid artery will often mark the lateral border of the thyroid gland.
- Bilateral neck assessment
  - Evaluate the neck for signs of lymphadenopathy in association with thyroid disease.
  - Beginning just below the mandible, scan from superior to inferior in transverse along the bilateral internal jugular veins and carotid arteries. Regions of the neck can be assessed and labeled accordingly (see Fig. 10-3).

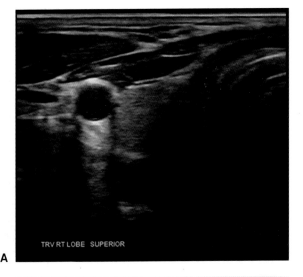

TRV RT LOBE SUPERIOR

A

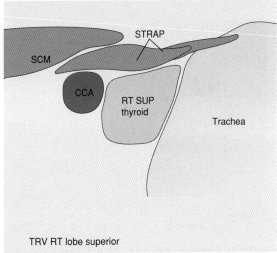

STRAP

SCM

CCA

RT SUP
thyroid

Trachea

B   TRV RT lobe superior

Figure 10-9. **Transverse superior right lobe. A, B: Superior right
thyroid lobe (RT SUP) with adjacent anatomy, including the
common carotid artery (CCA), strap muscles (STRAP), and the
sternocleidomastoid muscle (SCM).**

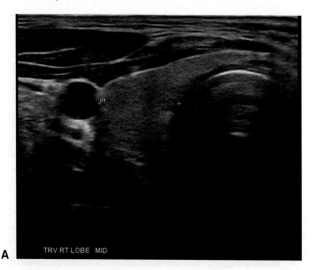

A   TRV RT LOBE MID

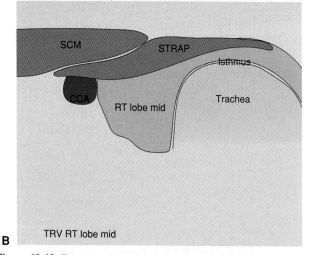

B   TRV RT lobe mid

Figure 10-10. Transverse mid right lobe. A, B: Transverse image of the mid right thyroid lobe with measurement of the thyroid width. In this image, the common carotid artery (CCA) can be seen laterally and the sternocleidomastoid muscle and strap muscles anteriorly. The trachea and thyroid isthmus are also noted.

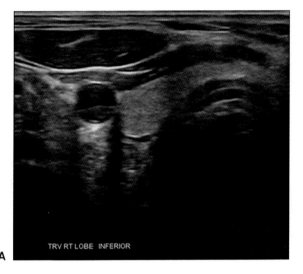

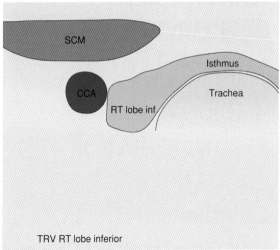

Figure 10-11. **Transverse inferior right lobe. A, B: Transverse image of the right inferior thyroid (RT LOBE INF) including the isthmus, trachea, common carotid artery (CCA), and the sternocleidomastoid muscle (SCM).**

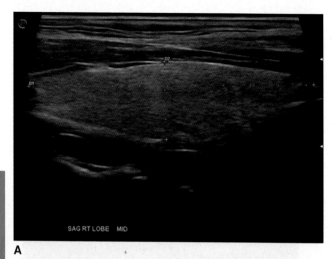

A

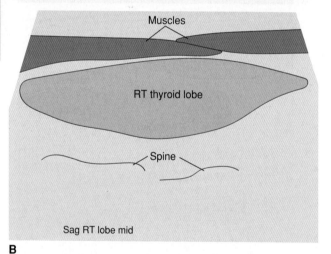

B

Figure 10-12. Longitudinal mid right lobe. A, B: Longitudinal right thyroid lobe (between *calipers*) with measurements.

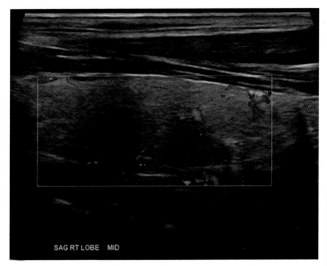

SAG RT LOBE   MID

Figure 10-13. Longitudinal mid right lobe with color Doppler.

- Document and measure any abnormal-appearing cervical lymph nodes in two orthogonal planes (see Essential Face and Neck Pathology in this chapter).
- Documentation of abnormalities[1]
  - Visualized thyroid abnormalities should be documented.
  - The location, size, number, and character of significant abnormalities should be documented, and measurements should be made in three dimensions.
  - In patients with numerous nodules in each lobe, measurements of all nodules are not necessary. The largest nodules or those with the most worrisome features should be selectively measured when multiple nodules are present.
  - Doppler analysis of lesions may be helpful.
  - Other abnormalities, such as venous thrombosis, should be documented.
- Additional images
  - Dual thyroid image
    - An image of both thyroid lobes can be used to assess the overall echogenicity of the thyroid and, in part, to compare the size of each lobe.

10. Neck and Face

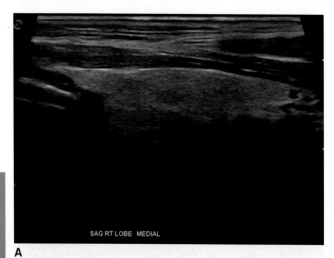

SAG RT LOBE MEDIAL

A

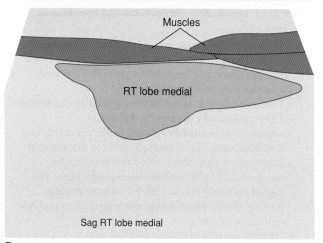

Muscles

RT lobe medial

Sag RT lobe medial

B

Figure 10-14. **Longitudinal right lobe medial. A, B:** Medial aspect of the right lobe.

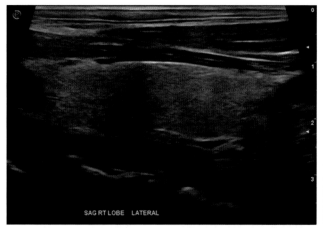

A

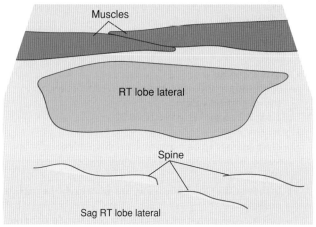

B

Figure 10-15. **Longitudinal right lobe lateral. A, B: Medial aspect of the right lobe.**

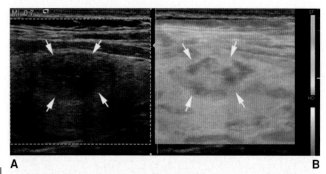

A   B

**Figure 10-16. Elastogram of a thyroid nodule. A: Representative
grayscale image of a hypoechoic indeterminate nodule (*arrows*).
B: Elastogram image shows the periphery of the nodule (*arrows*),
which has a red hue and constitutes the stiffer or harder (nonelastic)
component of the nodule. This mass was highly suspicious for
malignancy.** (Reprinted with permission from Siegel MJ, ed. *Pediatric
Sonography*. 4th ed. Philadelphia, PA: Wolters Kluwer Health/Lippincott
Williams & Wilkins; 2010.)

- Thyroid volume[2]
  - Some ultrasound machines contain capabilities of
    storing thyroid volume.
  - Thyroid volume = $L \times W \times H \times 0.529$
- Elastography[2]
  - Elastograms can be performed on thyroid lesions to
    assess for the presence of abnormal tissue stiffness
    (Fig. 10-16).
  - In theory, the stiffer the tissue, the more likely the mass is
    malignant.
  - Fine-needle aspiration remains the gold standard for the
    tissue characterization of thyroid lesions.
- Thyroidectomy patients:
  - Scan the entire neck, from just under the mandible to
    the clavicle bilaterally, especially in those patients with a
    history of thyroid cancer because there may be lingering
    lymphadenopathy.
- Parathyroid glands
  - Perform an assessment of the neck with Figure 10-2 in
    mind.

- If visualized, measure each parathyroid gland in two orthogonal planes.
- Cervical lymph nodes
  - Perform an assessment of the cervical lymph node chains with Figure 10-3 in mind.
  - If visualized, measure any abnormal-appearing cervical lymph nodes.
  - Label the regional lymph nodes, if warranted.
- Salivary glands[4]
  - Parotid glands
    - Transverse views are obtained by placing the transducer perpendicular and inferior to the earlobe.
    - Longitudinal views are obtained by placing the transducer anterior and parallel to the ear.
    - Color Doppler may be utilized to differentiate dilated ducts from vascular structures.
    - Hyperemia may indicate sialadenitis.
    - Sialolithiasis (salivary stones) will appear hyperechoic and may shadow.
  - Submandibular glands
    - The submandibular glands are evaluated by placing the transducer just under the mentum and angling the transducer coronally and sagittally.
    - Color Doppler may be utilized to differentiate dilated ducts from vascular structures.
    - Hyperemia may indicate sialadenitis.
    - Sialolithiasis (salivary stones) will appear hyperechoic and may shadow.
  - Sublingual glands
    - The sublingual glands are imaged with the transducer placed perpendicular and parallel to the submental mandible.

SCANNING TIPS

- When prominent, the esophagus may suggest the presence of a mass within the neck. It is often located posterior to the left thyroid lobe. Have the patient swallow to confirm the esophagus. Saliva will be seen passing through the esophagus.
- The bilateral longus colli muscles can be noted posterior to each thyroid lobe and may simulate a mass (**Fig. 10-17**).

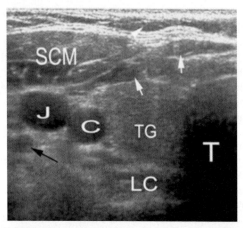

Figure 10-17. Longus colli muscle. A transverse section of the thyroid gland demonstrating the sternocleidomastoid muscle **(SCM)** beneath the subcutaneous fat (*white arrowhead*). The infrahyoid strap muscles lie deep to the fat and medial to the sternocleidomastoid muscle (*white arrows*). The jugular vein **(J)** and carotid artery **(C)** are prominent lateral boundaries defining the position of the thyroid gland **(TG)**. The longus colli muscle **(LC)** is seen deep to the gland, and the trachea **(T)** is the midline landmark.
(Reprinted with permission from Mancuso AA, ed. *Head and Neck Radiology*. 1st ed. Philadelphia, PA: Wolters Kluwer Health/Lippincott Williams & Wilkins; 2010.)

- A stand-off device or mounded gel may be warranted for superficial masses and for the assessment of the salivary glands.

NORMAL MEASUREMENTS OF THE NECK AND FACE[2]

- Thyroid
  - Lobes
    - Length = 4–6 cm
    - Anteroposterior = 1–2 cm
    - Transverse dimension = 2–3 cm
  - Isthmus = between 2 and 6 mm in thickness
  - Thyroid volume = L × W × H × 0.529
- Parathyroid
  - Parathyroid glands typically measure <5 mm in length.
- Normal lymph nodes

- Normal nodes measure <5 or 6 mm in the longest dimension, though they may measure up to 1 cm.

ESSENTIAL NECK AND FACE PATHOLOGY[2]

- Thyroid gland
  - Thyroid imaging, reporting, and data system (TI-RADS) calculator link: http://tiradscalculator.com/
    - The American College of Radiology released a white paper in 2018 on the use of TI-RADS in the clinical setting as a means of characterizing thyroid lesions detected with sonography and in order to prevent unnecessary biopsies.
  - Characteristics of benign thyroid nodules:
    - Extensive cystic components
    - Cysts <5 mm
    - Hyperechoic mass
    - "Eggshell" calcification surrounding the mass
  - Characteristics of malignant thyroid nodules:
    - Hypoechoic mass (possibly solitary)
    - Taller-than-wide shape
    - Solid mass with internal microcalcifications
    - Irregular margins
  - Graves disease (hyperthyroidism)
    - Clinical findings:
      - Bulging eyes
      - Heat intolerance
      - Nervousness
      - Weight loss
      - Hair loss
    - Sonographic findings:
      - Enlarged gland
      - Heterogeneous or diffusely hypoechoic echotexture (Fig. 10-18)
      - Thyroid inferno (increased vascularity)
  - Hashimoto thyroiditis (hypothyroidism)
    - Clinical findings:
      - Depression
      - Increased cold sensitivity
      - Elevated blood cholesterol levels
      - Slight weight gain
      - Puffy face and puffiness under the eyes

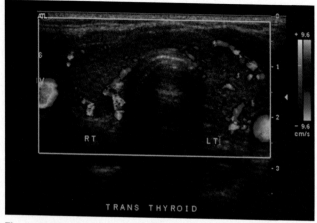

Figure 10-18. Graves disease. Transverse image of the thyroid demonstrating increased vascularity. The patient had clinical symptoms consistent with hyperthyroidism. (Reprinted with permission from Siegel MJ, ed. *Pediatric Sonography*. 5th ed. Philadelphia, PA: Wolters Kluwer; 2018.)

- Sonographic findings:
  - Mild enlargement of the gland initially
  - Heterogeneous echotexture **(Fig. 10-19)**
  - Numerous, ill-defined hypoechoic regions separated by fibrous bands
  - Increased vascularity
- Parathyroid glands
  - Parathyroid adenoma
    - Clinical findings:
      - Elevated serum calcium and PTH
      - Possible palpable mass
    - Sonographic findings:
      - Hypoechoic mass adjacent to the thyroid
- Other neck masses
  - Thyroglossal duct cyst
    - Clinical findings:
      - Palpable midline mass superior to the thyroid
    - Sonographic findings:
      - Anechoic or complex cyst within the midline of the neck superior to the thyroid

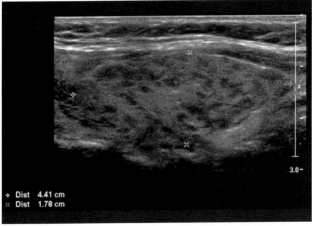

A

◆ Dist 4.41 cm
✖ Dist 1.78 cm

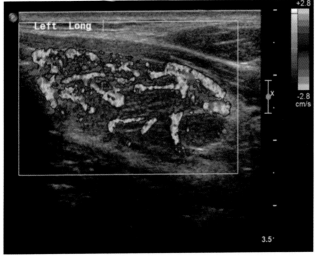

B

Figure 10-19. **Hashimoto thyroiditis. A: Longitudinal image of a heterogeneous thyroid gland. B: Increased vascularity is depicted with color Doppler.** (Reprinted with permission from Kawamura D, Nolan T, eds. *Abdomen and Superficial Structures.* 4th ed. Philadelphia, PA: Wolters Kluwer; 2017.)

- Branchial cleft cyst
  - Clinical findings:
    - ○ Palpable lateral neck mass
  - Sonographic findings:
    - ○ Anechoic mass
- Cervical lymphadenopathy
  - Clinical findings:
    - Possible palpable mass
  - Sonographic findings:
    - Node that measure >1 cm
    - Rounded shape or has irregular margins (Fig. 10-20)
    - Loss of echogenic hilum
    - Calcifications
    - Hyperemia may be present
- Salivary gland
  - Pleomorphic adenoma
    - Clinical findings:
      - ○ Enlargement of the parotid gland
    - Sonographic findings:
      - ○ Hypoechoic mass

WHERE ELSE TO LOOK

- Thyroid gland
  - Don't forget to scan the lateral neck for irregular-appearing lymph nodes.
- Parathyroid glands
  - Remember, there can be ectopic locations for parathyroid glands (see Fig. 10-2).
- Cervical lymphadenopathy
  - When a suspicious thyroid nodule is discovered, look carefully throughout the neck for enlarged or irregular-appearing lymph nodes.

IMAGE CORRELATION

- Malignant thyroid mass on CT (Fig. 10-21)

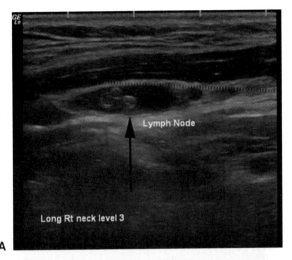

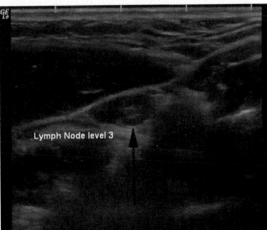

Figure 10-20. Abnormal appearing lymph node. Ultrasound
examination of the right lateral cervical lymph nodes shows an
abnormal right level III lymph node in the longitudinal (A) and
transverse (B) images. The arrows denote the abnormal lymph node.
(Reprinted with permission from Dimick JB, Upchurch GR, Sonnenday CJ,
eds. *Clinical Scenarios in Surgery.* 1st ed. Philadelphia, PA: Wolters Kluwer
Health/Lippincott Williams & Wilkins; 2012.)

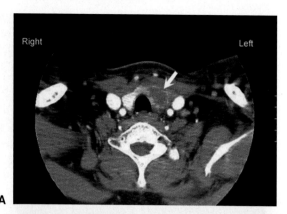

A

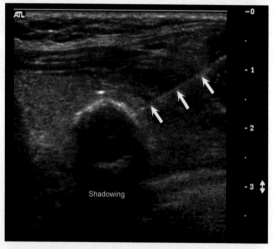

B

Figure 10-21. Follicular carcinoma. A: The computed tomography (CT) with contrast image demonstrates the sectional neck anatomy and a heterogeneous area beginning in the isthmus and extending throughout the left thyroid lobe arrow. B: The transverse sonogram of the left thyroid mass shows a diagonal line (*white arrows*) entering the image from the right, which is the biopsy needle used during a sonography-guided fine-needle aspiration biopsy. The cytology report diagnosed follicular carcinoma. (Reprinted with permission from Kawamura D, Nolan T, eds. *Abdomen and Superficial Structures*. 4th ed. Philadelphia, PA: Wolters Kluwer; 2017.)

REFERENCES

1. AIUM practice parameters for the performance of ultrasound examinations of the head and neck. https://www.aium.org/resources/guidelines/headNeck.pdf. Accessed September 4, 2018.
2. Penny SM, ed. *Examination Review for Ultrasound: Abdomen & Obstetrics and Gynecology.* 2nd ed. Philadelphia, PA: Wolters Kluwer; 2018:189–201.
3. Kawamura DM, Nolan TD, eds. *Diagnostic Medical Sonography: Abdomen and Superficial Structures.* 4th ed. Philadelphia, PA: Wolters Kluwer; 2018:421–454.
4. Seigel MJ, ed. *Pediatric Sonography.* 4th ed. Philadelphia, PA: Wolters Kluwer; 2011:118–163.

CHAPTER 11

Breast

INTRODUCTION

Sonography is an outstanding adjunct to mammography in the characterization of breast lesions. Oftentimes, sonography immediately follows the mammographic detection of a worrisome lesion or suspicious finding. Sonography can also be used as an initial imaging tool for young women prior to receiving their earliest screening mammogram. This chapter will provide a brief overview of breast imaging. The sonographer should have a thorough understanding of the benefits and limitations of sonography. Protocols for breast sonography may vary among institutions. Guidelines that have been established for breast imaging in each institution must be carefully followed in order to provide each patient with standardized, and yet case-specific optimal sonographic imaging.

AIUM AND ACR RECOMMENDATION FOR SONOGRAPHY OF THE BREAST[1]

- Assess the breast in the following manner:
  - Evaluate and sonographically characterize palpable masses and other breast-related signs and/or symptoms.
  - Evaluate abnormalities identified on other imaging modalities, including mammography and breast magnetic resonance imaging (MRI).
  - Initially assess palpable breast masses in patients <30 yrs of age and in lactating women.
  - Evaluate for breast implant complications.
  - Assist in the sonographic guidance of breast biopsies and axillary lymph nodes, interventional procedures, and treatment planning for radiation therapy.
  - Provide a screening tool, in conjunction with mammography, for occult cancers in certain populations.

ESSENTIAL ANATOMY AND PHYSIOLOGY OF THE BREAST[2–4]

- Anatomy and physiology of the breast
  - The breast is an exocrine organ, with the primary function of producing milk following childbirth.
  - The breast has three major portions: the skin, the subcutaneous fat, and the glandular parenchyma of the breast, which is the functional component and the location of most cancers (**Fig. 11-1**). The breast may also be divided into three zones: premammary, mammary, and retromammary.
  - The tail of the breast, or its axillary process, extends toward the axilla.
  - The glandular breast consists of 15–20 segments or lobes that are separated by connective tissue. These lobes can be divided further into lobules.
  - Five to ten major collecting milk or lactiferous ducts radiate from the nipple into the lobules and work to drain the breast of milk in the direction of the nipple.
  - The functional, glandular unit of the breast is the terminal duct lobular unit.
  - Cooper suspensory ligaments provide support to the breast.
  - Developmental changes of the breast occur during a woman's life:
    - In the young girl, with the production of estrogen by the ovaries, the glandular portion of the breast increases.
    - The glandular portion of the breast is thick in a young woman compared to the fat component.
    - An increase of fatty components and more functional tissue occurs during pregnancy and lactation.
    - As the female advances in age, fatty components increase.
  - Fibrocystic breasts are composed of scattered fibrotic and cystic areas and are a common variant in childbearing ages.
  - Atrophy of the breast during and after menopause results in an increase in fatty components, while the functional component decreases in size, a variant that may be referred to as fatty breast.

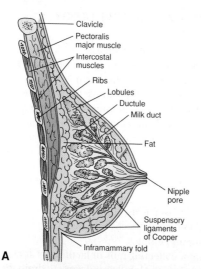

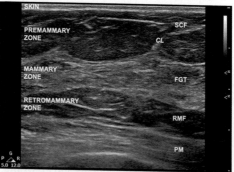

Figure 11-1. Anatomy of the breast. A: Sagittal schematic of the breast. **B:** Sonogram of the breast demonstrates the skin layer, the subcutaneous fat (SCF), and Copper ligament (CL) within the premammary zone; fibroglandular tissue (FGT) within the mammary zone; retromammary fat (RMF) within the retromammary zone; and the pectoralis major muscle (PM). The mammary zone is encased within the anterior and posterior mammary fascial planes.

(Image A reprinted with permission from Jensen S, ed. *Nursing Health Assessment*. 1st ed. Philadelphia, PA: Wolters Kluwer Health/Lippincott Williams & Wilkins; 2010; Image B reprinted with permission from Kawamura D, Nolan T, eds. *Abdomen and Superficial Structures*. 4th ed. Philadelphia, PA: Wolters Kluwer; 2017.)

11. Breast

PATIENT PREPARATION FOR SONOGRAPHY OF THE BREAST

- No patient preparation is typically required for a sonogram of the breast.

SUGGESTED EQUIPMENT[1]

- Equipment includes a linear array transducer with a center frequency of at least 12 MHz or higher with electronically adjustable focal zones.
- A stand-off device or mounded gel may be required for imaging of superficial lesions.

CLINICAL INVESTIGATION FOR SONOGRAPHY OF THE BREAST

- Laboratory values are listed in **Table 11-1**.
- Evaluate prior imaging reports and images including previous sonograms, mammography, CT, MRI, radiography, and any other appropriate tests.
- The BI-RADS US categories are provided in **Table 11-2** as a basic overview.
- Critical clinical history questions related to the breast
  - Is there any family history of breast cancers or tumors? *When appropriate, this is a helpful initial question to be asked before you begin scanning. If so, further inquire about when, and if found in a relative, which relative (e.g., mother, aunt, etc.).*
  - Do you have a mass that you can feel? *The patient may be able to palpate the mass herself. If so, have her indicate the location with her finger or her hand.*
  - How long has the mass been there? *This is an important question with regard to aging the mass.*
  - Is the mass mobile or stationary? *In theory, a mobile mass, or one that can be pushed around in the breast, is likely benign. A mass that is nonmobile or stiff is likely malignant.*

Table 11-1	LAB FINDINGS AND POSSIBLE ASSOCIATED BREAST PATHOLOGY
LAB FINDING	**POTENTIAL PATHOLOGY**
↑ WBC (leukocytosis)	Mastitis

11. Breast

Table 11-2	BI-RADS US CATEGORIES AND BASIC OVERVIEW[5]

CATEGORY	BASIC OVERVIEW
Category 0: Incomplete	Patient requires additional imaging
Category 1: Negative	Essentially 0% likelihood of malignancy
Category 2: Benign	Essentially 0% likelihood of malignancy
Category 3: Probably benign	<0% but ≤2% likelihood of malignancy
Category 4: Suspicious Category 4A: Low suspicion Category 4B: Moderate suspicion Category 4C: High suspicion	>2% but <95% likelihood of malignancy
Category 5: Highly suggestive of malignancy	≥95% likelihood of malignancy
Category 6: Known biopsy-proven malignancy	N/A

- In what position do you feel the mass the best? *A mass may only be felt by the patient in the upright position, and thus scanning in that position may be helpful.*
- Are you having any nipple discharge? *Any nipple discharge and the color of the discharge should be reported to the radiologist.*
- Is there discoloration of the skin? *Discoloration or dimpling of the skin is a possible finding with infection and/or cancer, and should be reported to the radiologist.*
- Are there any lumps in the armpit? *A palpable mass in the armpit may be a sign of metastasis to an axillary lymph node.*
- Are you breastfeeding? *Breastfeeding can significantly improve the visualization of the ducts. Also, some breast masses are more common during lactation.*

NORMAL SONOGRAPHIC DESCRIPTION
OF THE BREAST[1,6]

- Subcutaneous fat typically consists of medium gray echoes and is more hypoechoic than fibroglandular tissue, which is light gray.
- Dense glandular tissue is often defined sonographically as round, oval, or elongated hypoechoic regions surrounded by an echogenic background **(Fig. 11-2)**.
- Fatty tissue appears as hypoechoic tissue surrounded and delineated by echogenic ligaments **(Fig. 11-3)**.
- Heterogeneous breast tissue demonstrates a mixture of hypoechoic and echogenic areas.
- Lactiferous ducts may be seen as linear, branching tubular channels within the breast tissue.
- The nipple may simulate a mass or produce a significant shadow.
- Ribs will be equally spaced round structures in the far field in the cross section and will produce a shadow **(Fig. 11-4)**.

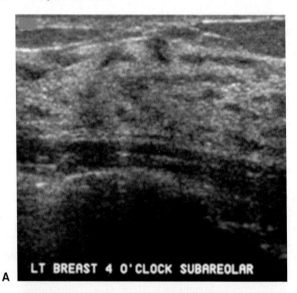

LT BREAST 4 O'CLOCK SUBAREOLAR

A

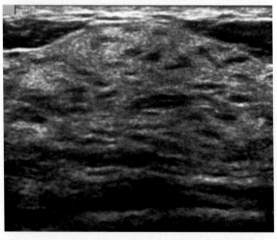

B

Figure 11-2. **Dense breast tissue. A: Dense breast tissue often appears as round, oval, or elongated hypoechoic areas in an echogenic background. B: A fibrous ridge of tissue is noted in this image.** (Reprinted with permission from Cardenosa G, ed. *Breast Imaging Companion*. 4th ed. Philadelphia, PA: Wolters Kluwer; 2017.)

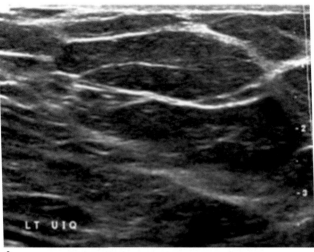

A

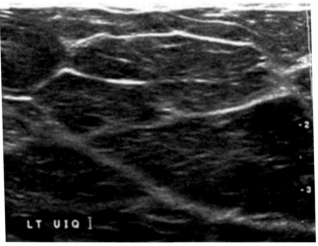

B

Figure 11-3. **Fatty breast tissue. A, B: Two images of fatty tissue, which is depicted sonographically as hypoechoic tissue surrounded and delineated by echogenic ligaments.** (Reprinted with permission from Cardenosa G, ed. *Breast Imaging Companion*. 4th ed. Philadelphia, PA: Wolters Kluwer; 2017.)

11. Breast

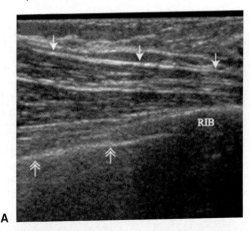

A

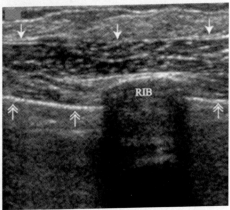

B

Figure 11-4. Pectoralis muscles and ribs. A: The pectoral muscle is hypoechoic. In this orientation of the transducer, parallel echogenic striations are noted in the substance of the muscle. The deep pectoral fascia (*arrows*) serves to delineate the pectoral muscle from overlying breast tissue. The pleura is seen as an echogenic line (*double-headed arrows*) deep to the pectoral muscle. B: The pectoral muscle is hypoechoic. The deep pectoral fascia (*arrows*) serves to delineate the pectoral muscle from overlying breast tissue. The rib is associated with shadowing that interrupts visualization of the pleura (*double-headed arrows*). (Reprinted with permission from Cardenosa G, ed. *Breast Imaging Companion*. 4th ed. Philadelphia, PA: Wolters Kluwer; 2017.)

SUGGESTED PROTOCOL FOR SONOGRAPHY OF THE BREAST[1,6]

- The patient should be placed in a position that minimizes the thickness of the portion of the breast being evaluated, which often is in a slight posterior contralateral oblique position **(Fig. 11-5)**. Positioning may also be correlated to mammographic images **(Fig. 11-6)**.
- The ipsilateral arm should be raised and placed behind the patient's head.
- The requested region should be imaged in at least two perpendicular projections—that is to say, either transverse and longitudinal or radial and antiradial **(Fig. 11-7)**.
- Clock-face notation should be provided, as well as distance from the nipple. Do not measure from the areola **(Fig. 11-8)**.
- A quadrant location and 1-2-3 and A-B-C annotation may be required by some institutions **(Fig. 11-9)**.
- The time gain compensation should be adjusted in order to differentiate fatty tissue from glandular tissue and the focal zone should be placed at the depth of identifiable lesions.

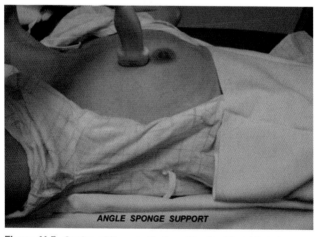

ANGLE SPONGE SUPPORT

Figure 11-5. Supine-oblique patient positioning. The side to be examined is elevated by a foam support and the patient's arm is positioned near the head. This contralateral oblique position helps flatten the breast tissue over the chest. (Reprinted with permission from Kawamura D, Lunsford B, eds. *Abdomen and Superficial Structures.* 3rd ed. Philadelphia, PA: Wolters Kluwer Health/Lippincott Williams & Wilkins; 2012.)

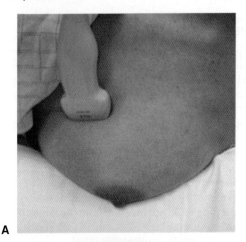

A

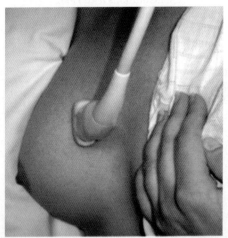

B

Figure 11-6. Positioning for sonography of the breast. A: Upright positioning can be used to compare the sonography location of a mass to the mammographic craniocaudal view. B: Decubital positioning, in this case, is used to access the medial breast to compare relative mass location with the MLO or 90° lateral mammographic views. The patient can be rolled to better access the lateral breast. (Reprinted with permission from Kawamura D, Lunsford B, eds. *Abdomen and Superficial Structures.* 3rd ed. Philadelphia, PA: Wolters Kluwer Health/Lippincott Williams & Wilkins; 2012.)

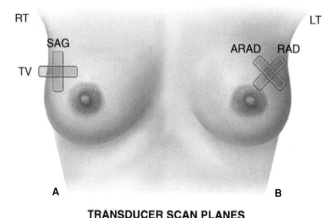

TRANSDUCER SCAN PLANES

Figure 11-7. Perpendicular scan planes. A: Schematic of traditional sagittal (SAG) and transverse (TV) scan planes. B: Radial (RAD) and antiradial (ARAD) scan planes. (Reprinted with permission from Kawamura D, Lunsford B, eds. *Abdomen and Superficial Structures.* 3rd ed. Philadelphia, PA: Wolters Kluwer Health/Lippincott Williams & Wilkins; 2012.)

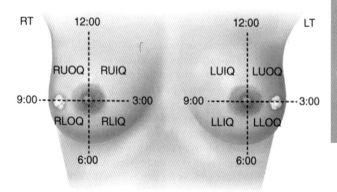

QUADRANT AND CLOCK-FACE ANNOTATION

Figure 11-8. Quadrant and clock-face annotation. Some institutions will require clock-face and/or quadrant annotation. (Reprinted with permission from Kawamura D, Lunsford B, eds. *Abdomen and Superficial Structures.* 3rd ed. Philadelphia, PA: Wolters Kluwer Health/Lippincott Williams & Wilkins; 2012.)

11. Breast

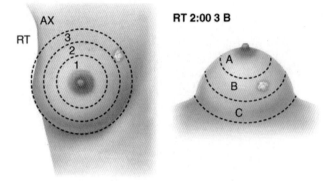

"1-2-3 A-B-C" ANNOTATION

Figure 11-9. 1-2-3-A-B-C annotation. Some institutions may require this format of labeling. 1 depicts the inner third of the breast, 2 is the mid third of the breast, while 3 is the outer third of the breast. A is the anterior third of the breast, B is the middle third of the breast, while C is the posterior third of the breast. (Reprinted with permission from Kawamura D, Lunsford B, eds. *Abdomen and Superficial Structures.* 3rd ed. Philadelphia, PA: Wolters Kluwer Health/Lippincott Williams & Wilkins; 2012.)

- The depth should be deep enough in order to include the pectoralis muscle.
- If possible, the transducer should be manipulated with one hand, while the fingers of the other hand are simultaneously moved back and forth at the leading edge of the transducer in order to correlate what is being imaged with what is being felt.
- If a suspected abnormality is identified in one plane, the transducer should be rotated 90 degrees in order to confirm the presence of the abnormality in two planes (**Fig. 11-10**).
- The sonographer should scan completely through a mass, noting the borders carefully for signs of irregular margins.
- A measureable abnormality should be documented in images that are obtained with measurements and without measurements in two perpendicular projections.
- Masses behind the nipple may require the peripheral compression technique or the rolled-nipple technique (**Figs. 11-11 and 11-12**).

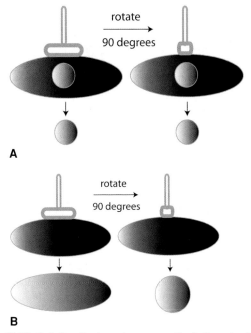

Figure 11-10. Rotating the transducer correctly. A: If a potential lesion is identified, it is important to rotate the transducer over the area. A true lesion remains discrete (oval, round, or irregular) as the transducer is rotated. **B:** Oblong breast tissue bundles are intercalated within the skeleton provided by Cooper ligaments. If a bundle is imaged in cross section it may appear mass-like; however, as the transducer is rotated over this area the pseudomass elongates, becomes less apparent, and often fuses with the surrounding tissue. (Reprinted with permission from Cardenosa G, ed. *Breast Imaging Companion*. 4th ed. Philadelphia, PA: Wolters Kluwer; 2017.)

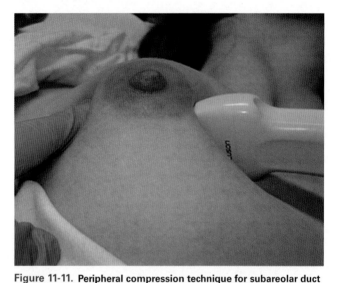

Figure 11-11. Peripheral compression technique for subareolar duct evaluation. The transducer is oriented in a radial plane along the axis of the duct to be examined. The nonscanning hand is placed on the opposite side of the breast to provide counter pressure. The transducer is angled by applying pressure to the peripheral edge of the transducer. This maneuver brings the subareolar duct into a scan plane more parallel to the transducer. Sliding the transducer toward the nipple follows the duct. (Reprinted with permission from Kawamura D, Nolan T, eds. *Abdomen and Superficial Structures.* 4th ed. Philadelphia, PA: Wolters Kluwer; 2017.)

- Color Doppler should be employed to provide an analysis of the vascularity of the lesion.
- Elastography, which essentially characterizes a mass based on tissue stiffness, can also be utilized. In theory, the stiffer the tissue, the more likely the mass is malignant (**Fig. 11-13**). However, manufacturer guidelines and settings vary, and thus training in the use of elastography and interpretation of elastograms in the clinical setting is warranted to provide optimal patient care.

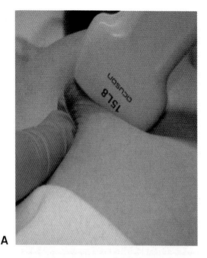

A

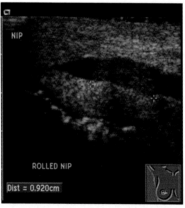

B

Figure 11-12. **Rolled-nipple technique. A: The transducer is placed along the nipple and breast in a radial plane parallel to the long axis of the excretory and subareolar duct. The index finger of the sonographer's nonscanning hand is placed on the opposite side of the nipple. Light transducer pressure is applied to roll the nipple over the index finger. This maneuver allows a subareolar duct to be imaged as it passes through the nipple to evaluate for an intraductal mass. B: The sonogram shows a nipple adenoma within a dilated excretory duct using the rolled-nipple technique.** (Reprinted with permission from Kawamura D, Nolan T, eds. *Abdomen and Superficial Structures*. 4th ed. Philadelphia, PA: Wolters Kluwer; 2017.)

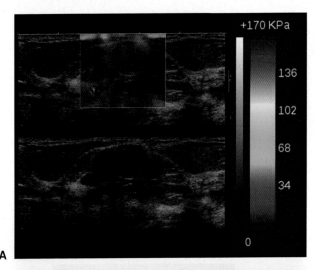

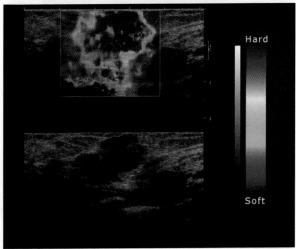

Figure 11-13. Shear-wave elastograms. A: 2D image (lower image) and elastogram of a benign mass. B: This multilobulated lesion displays hard (stiff) elastic features, typical of a malignant mass. (Reprinted with permission from Kawamura D, Nolan T, eds. *Abdomen and Superficial Structures*. 4th ed. Philadelphia, PA: Wolters Kluwer; 2017.)

SCANNING TIPS[3]

- The sonographer should learn more about mammography and how to correctly view mammograms so that he or she can better understand the location of masses **(Figs. 11-14 and 11-15)**.
- The patient should indicate the area of a palpable lesion with her finger or hand.
- Upright imaging may be helpful, especially if that is the position in which a palpable mass is best felt by the patient.
- Transducer pressure that is too light can cause simulated shadowing, while scanning with too much pressure can result in obscuring underlying lesions.
- A stand-off pad should be used to improve the visualization of superficial masses. Mounded gel can also be utilized.
- Microcalcifications demonstrated on a mammogram may not be seen sonographically.
- Vocal fremitus may be utilized as well. To do this, have the patient hum "eee" while scanning with color Doppler or power Doppler **(Fig. 11-16)**. Certain abnormal tissues and masses will be devoid of Doppler signals.

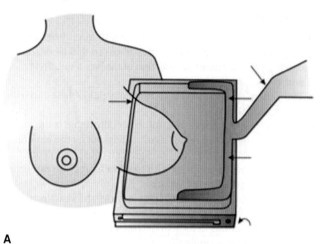

A

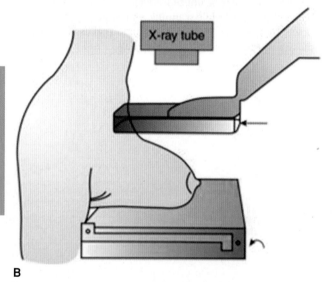

X-ray tube

B

Figure 11-14. Mammographic projections. A: Mediolateral projection (MLO). B: Craniocaudal projection (CC). (Reprinted with permission from Smith WL, ed. *Radiology 101*. 4th ed. Philadelphia, PA: Wolters Kluwer Health/Lippincott Williams & Wilkins; 2013.)

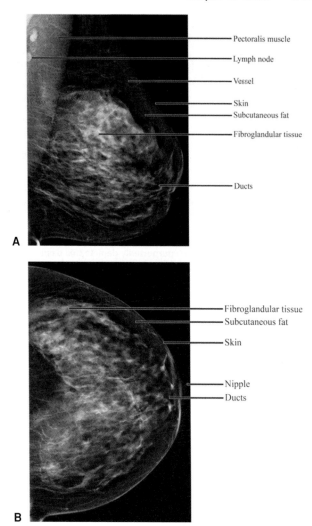

A

- Pectoralis muscle
- Lymph node
- Vessel
- Skin
- Subcutaneous fat
- Fibroglandular tissue
- Ducts

B

- Fibroglandular tissue
- Subcutaneous fat
- Skin
- Nipple
- Ducts

Figure 11-15. Normal mammogram. A: Left breast mediolateral oblique (MLO) digital mammogram. Normal. B: Left breast craniocaudal (CC) digital mammogram. Normal. (Reprinted with permission from Smith WL, ed. *Radiology 101*. 4th ed. Philadelphia, PA: Wolters Kluwer Health/Lippincott Williams & Wilkins; 2013.)

11. Breast

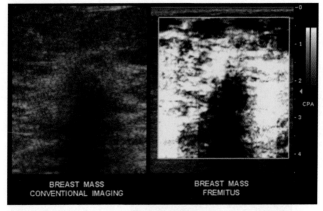

Figure 11-16. Vocal fremitus. Conventional two-dimensional sonogram on the left and on the right, power Doppler reveals an area devoid of color, which purportedly depicts this tissue as being more dense and thus increases the likelihood of an area of abnormal tissue. (Reprinted with permission from Kawamura D, Lunsford B, eds. *Abdomen and Superficial Structures*. 3rd ed. Philadelphia, PA: Wolters Kluwer Health/Lippincott Williams & Wilkins; 2012.)

NORMAL MEASUREMENTS OF THE BREAST

● Skin covering the breast typically measures not more than 2 mm

ESSENTIAL BREAST PATHOLOGY[3,6]

● Benign features of solid breast masses:
  ● Hyperechoic mass
  ● Well-circumscribed margins
  ● Wider than tall
  ● Bilobulated or trilobulated
  ● Thin echogenic pseudocapsule
● Malignant feature of solid breast masses:
  ● Markedly hypoechoic
  ● Speculated borders
  ● Taller than wide
  ● Angular or indistinct margins
  ● Irregular echogenic rim around the mass
  ● Posterior shadowing
  ● Microlobulations

- Duct extension
- Branch pattern
- Calcifications within the mass
- Possible posterior enhancement
- Breast cyst **(Fig. 11-17)**
  - Clinical findings:
    - Possible palpable mass
  - Sonographic findings:
    - Anechoic mass
    - Posterior enhancement
    - Well-circumscribed mass
    - Thin, echogenic capsule
- Fibroadenoma—a common solid benign breast mass **(Fig. 11-18)**
  - Clinical findings:
    - Possible palpable mass
  - Sonographic findings:
    - Hypoechoic mass
    - Well-circumscribed margins
    - Wider than tall
    - Bilobulated or trilobulated
    - Thin, echogenic pseudocapsule
- Infiltrative ductal carcinoma **(Fig. 11-19)**
  - Clinical findings:
    - Possible palpable mass
    - Skin dimpling
    - Nipple discharge
    - Red, swollen breast with skin edema ("peau d'orange")
    - Possible family history
  - Sonographic findings:
    - Markedly hypoechoic
    - Speculated borders
    - Taller than wide
    - Angular or indistinct margins
    - Irregular echogenic rim around the mass
    - Posterior shadowing
    - Microlobulations
    - Duct extension
    - Branch pattern
    - Calcifications within the mass
    - Possible posterior enhancement

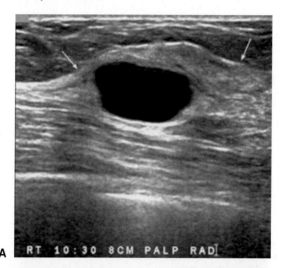

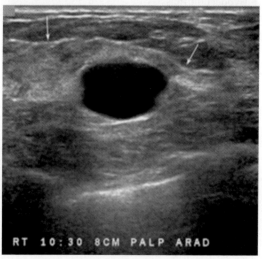

Figure 11-17. Breast cyst. A, B: Orthogonal ultrasound images of an anechoic mass with circumscribed margins and posterior acoustic enhancement in a fibrous ridge (*arrows*) of breast tissue. (Reprinted with permission from Cardenosa G, ed. *Breast Imaging Companion.* 4th ed. Philadelphia, PA: Wolters Kluwer; 2017.)

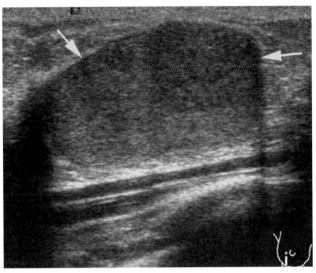

Figure 11-18. Fibroadenoma. A well-circumscribed hypoechoic solid mass corresponding with a palpable mass (*arrows*). (Reprinted with permission from Smith WL, ed. *Radiology 101*. 4th ed. Philadelphia, PA: Wolters Kluwer Health/Lippincott Williams & Wilkins; 2013.)

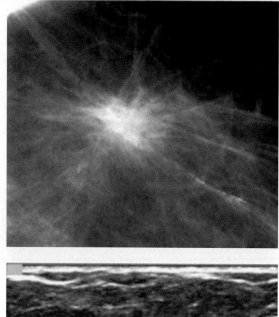

A

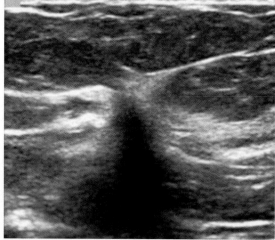

B

Figure 11-19. Ductal carcinoma. A: Mammogram image of a ductal carcinoma. B: Corresponding mass demonstrated with sonography.
(Reprinted with permission from Cardenosa G, ed. *Breast Imaging Companion.* 4th ed. Philadelphia, PA: Wolters Kluwer; 2017.)

WHERE ELSE TO LOOK

- The associated axilla should also be examined if a suspicious lesion is identified for associated lymphadenopathy, as well as the remaining breast tissue.
- The axilla should also be examined in cases of ruptured implants.

IMAGE CORRELATION

- MRI of the breast **(Fig. 11-20)**

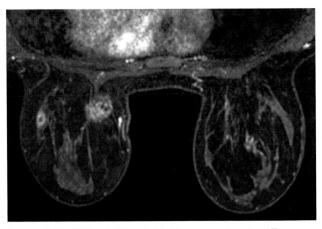

Figure 11-20. MRI, axial T1-weighted image, postcontrast. Two masses with heterogeneous enhancement are imaged at this level. The medial lesion is further characterized by spiculated margins and correlates with the site of the patient's known, screen-detected invasive ductal carcinoma. The lateral lesion at this level is the more anterior of the two masses seen laterally in the MIP image and demonstrates rim enhancement. (Reprinted with permission from Cardenosa G, ed. *Clinical Breast Imaging: The Essentials.* 1st ed. Philadelphia, PA: Wolters Kluwer; 2014.)

11. Breast

REFERENCES

1. ACR practice parameters for the performance of a breast ultrasound examination. https://www.acr.org/~/media/ACR/Files/Practice-Parameters/US-Breast.pdf. Accessed October 18, 2018.
2. Gibbs R, Karlan BY, Haney AF, Nygaard IE, eds. *Danforth's Obstetrics and Gynecology*. 10th ed. Philadelphia: Wolters Kluwer; 2008:932–958.
3. Sanders R, Hall-Terracciano B, eds. *Clinical Sonography: A Practical Guide*. 5th ed. Philadelphia: Wolters Kluwer; 2016:713–733.
4. Curry RA, Tempkin BB, eds. *Sonography: Introduction to Normal Structure and Function*. 4th ed. St. Louis, Missouri: Elsevier; 2015:519–528.
5. ACR BI-RADS ATLAS—breast ultrasound. https://www.acr.org/media/ACR/Files/RADS/BI-RADS/US-Reporting.pdf. Accessed October 19, 2018.
6. Cardenosa G, ed. *Breast Imaging Companion*. 4th ed. Philadelphia: Wolters Kluwer; 2017:103–129.

CHAPTER 12

Infant Hips, Neonatal Brain, and Neonatal Spine

INTRODUCTION

Abdominal sonographers may occasionally be required to perform additional sonographic examinations such as infant hip sonograms, neonatal brain sonograms, and sonograms of the neonatal spine. This chapter provides a summary of these examinations, including a suggested protocol, images, and an abbreviated overview of the most common pathologies one might encounter.

AIUM AND ACR RECOMMENDATION FOR SONOGRAPHY OF INFANT HIPS, NEONATAL BRAIN, AND NEONATAL SPINE

- Infant hips[1]:
  - A sonogram of the infant hip is often indicated when developmental dysplasia of the hip (DDH) is strongly suspected, especially when the following risk factors are present:
    - Frank breech presentation
    - History of a parent and/or sibling with DDH
    - Hip instability is present on physical examination
    - The infant has a neuromuscular condition that predisposes him or her to DDH
    - Oligohydramnios or other intrauterine causes of abnormal posturing
- Neonatal brain[2]:
  - Indications for a neonatal and infant brain sonogram include, but are not limited to, the following:

- Evaluation for hemorrhage or parenchymal abnormalities
- Evaluation for hydrocephalus
- Evaluation for signs of vascular disorders
- Evaluation for possible or suspected hypoxic–ischemic encephalopathy
- Follow-up of patients on hypothermia, extracorporeal membrane oxygenation, and other support machines
- Evaluation for signs/symptoms of central nervous disorders
- Evaluation of trauma
- Evaluation for craniosynostosis
- Follow-up or assessment of previously documented abnormalities, including those identified during a prenatal sonogram
- Screening before a surgical procedure

- Neonatal spine[3]:
  - Indications for a neonatal spine sonogram include, but are not limited to, the following:
    - External spinal signs suggestive of a spinal dysraphism or spinal cord tethering such as:
      - Midline or paramedian masses
      - Midline skin discoloration
      - Skin tags
      - Hair tuffs
      - Hemangiomas
      - Sacral dimples (small or deep)
        - Higher suspicion for occult lesions occurs with sacral dimples in which the base of dimple is not visualized, if it is located >2.5 cm above the anus, or is seen in combination with the above listed skin abnormalities.
    - Presence of caudal regression syndrome and anal atresia or stenosis
    - Evaluation of other suspected cord abnormalities including diastematomyelia, hydromyelia, and syringomyelia
    - Detection of hematoma following trauma, infection, or hemorrhage following prior instrumentation such as a lumbar puncture, or posttraumatic cerebrospinal fluid (CSF) leakage

- Visualization of blood products within the spinal canal in patients with intracranial hemorrhage
- Postoperative follow-up assessment of spinal surgeries

ESSENTIAL ANATOMY AND PHYSIOLOGY OF THE INFANT HIP, NEONATAL BRAIN, AND NEONATAL SPINE

- Anatomy and physiology of the infant hip[4]:
  - The hip bone is composed of the ilium, ischium, and pubis.
  - The infant hip joint is a ball-and-socket joint, with the femoral head normally resting within the acetabulum of the pelvic bone (Fig. 12-1).
  - The newborn hip is mostly cartilaginous, which allows for the sonographic assessment of the relationship between the femoral head and the acetabulum.
  - DDH is a congenital anomaly in which the newborn suffers from a shallow hip socket.
  - As a result of DDH, the newborn hip can be referred to as subluxed, which is defined as partially dislocated. It can also be completely dislocated or dislocatable upon physical examination (Fig. 12-2).
  - It is thought that perhaps circulating maternal hormones influence the laxity of fetal ligaments, thus possibly predisposing some newborns to hips that are either subluxable or dislocatable.
  - Fetal malposition, such as breech, and oligohydramnios greatly increase the likelihood of an infant suffering from DDH.
- Anatomy and physiology of the neonatal brain:
  - Anatomy:
    - Fontanelles:
      - Sonography utilizes the fontanelles to evaluate the infant brain:
        - The most common fontanelle utilized is the anterior fontanelle (Fig. 12-3).
        - Other fontanelles include posterior, mastoidal, and sphenoidal.
    - The two main portions of the brain are the cerebrum and the cerebellum, which are separated by a fold of dura mater referred to as the tentorium.

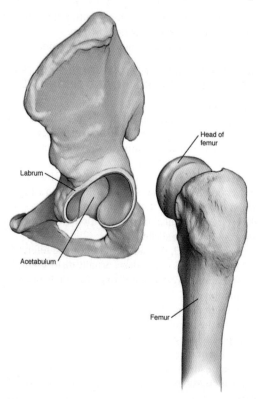

Figure 12-1. Basic anatomy of the hip joint. (Reprinted with permission from Flynn JM, Sankar WN, Wiesel SW, eds. *Operative Techniques in Pediatric Orthapaedic Surgery.* 2nd ed. Philadelphia, PA: Wolters Kluwer; 2016.)

○ Cerebrum:
  – The cerebrum is the largest superiorly positioned portion of the brain.
  – It can be separated into right and left hemispheres by the falx cerebri.
  – It is composed of an anterior frontal lobe, superior and laterally located paired parietal lobes, paired temporal lobes that are located inferior and lateral, and an occipital lobe that is posterior in location.

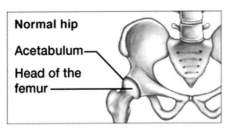

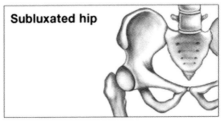

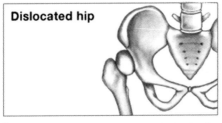

Figure 12-2. Developmental dysplasia of the hip. In developmental dysplasia of the hip, flattening of the acetabulum prevents the head of the femur from rotating adequately. The child's hip may be unstable, subluxated (partially dislocated), or completely dislocated. (Reprinted with permission from Penny S, ed. *Examination Review for Ultrasound: Abdomen and Obstetrics and Gynecology.* 2nd ed. Philadelphia, PA: Wolters Kluwer; 2017.)

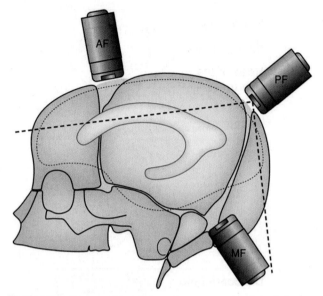

Figure 12-3. Sonographic windows for sonography of the infant brain. The anterior fontanelle (AF) is the most commonly utilized window, while the posterior fontanelle (PF) and mastoid fontanelle (MF) can also provide additional views. (Adapted with permission of American Society of Neuroradiology, from Correa F, Enriquez G, Rossello J, et al. Posterior fontanelle sonography: An acoustics window into the neonatal brain. *AJNR Am J Neuroradiol.* 2004;25(7):1274–1282. Permission conveyed through Copyright Clearance Center, Inc.)

- – The right and left cerebral hemispheres are connected by a band of tissue referred to as the corpus callosum.
- – The right and left lateral ventricles are located within the hemispheres respectively.
- – The cerebrum of the premature newborn may lack the normally demonstrated sulci and gyri of the full-term newborn.
- ○ Cerebellum:
  - – The cerebellum is the smaller posterior and inferiorly positioned part of the brain.
  - – It consists of a right and left hemisphere, connected in the midline by a structure referred to as the cerebellar vermis.

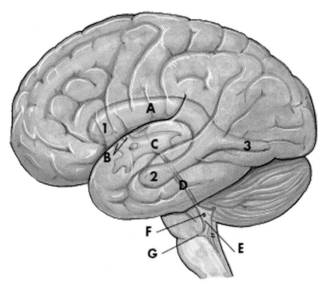

Figure 12-4. Lateral or sagittal anatomy of the ventricles of the brain. (A) Lateral ventricle: 1-Anterior horn; 2-Inferior horn; 3-Posterior horn, (B) Interventricular foramen (Monro), (C) Third ventricle, (D) Cerebral aqueduct, (E) Fourth ventricle, (F) Lateral foramen (Luschka), (G) Medial foramen (Magendie). (Reprinted with permission from Anatomical Chart Company. *Rapid Review Anatomy Reference Guide.* 3rd ed. Philadelphia, PA: Lippincott Williams & Wilkins; 2010.)

○ The ventricular system:
– The ventricles of the brain contain CSF, which is produced by choroid plexus that is mostly located in the bilateral lateral ventricles **(Fig. 12-4).** There are two lateral ventricles, one third ventricle, and one fourth ventricle.
– Lateral ventricles
■ The lateral ventricles are located within the right or left hemisphere, and each consists of a frontal horn, body, trigone or atrium, temporal or inferior horn, and occipital horn.
■ They contain the majority of choroid plexus, which is located in the atrium or trigone.

12. Pediatrics

- Third ventricle:
  - The third ventricle is located in the midline of the brain and linked to each lateral ventricle by the foramina of Monro.
  - The interthalamic adhesion travels through the third ventricle and may be readily noted when the third ventricle is distended with CSF.
- Fourth ventricle:
  - The fourth ventricle is connected to the third ventricle via the cerebral aqueduct (aqueduct of Sylvius).
  - It is located in the midline anterior to the cerebellar vermis.

○ Cisterna magna:
  - The cisterna magna is the largest cistern of the brain.
  - It is located posterior to the cerebellum.

○ Cavum septum pellucidum (CSP):
  - The CSP is a normal midline cystic brain structure that appears much more prominent in the neonatal brain.
  - The CSP is located between the frontal horns of the lateral ventricles, superior to the third ventricle and inferior to the corpus callosum (**Fig. 12-5**).
  - The posterior extension of the CSP within the premature brain is referred to as the cavum vergae.
  - The CSP closes from posterior to anterior as the brain matures.

○ Thalamus:
  - The lobes of the thalamus are located below each cerebral lobe and form the lateral borders of the third ventricle.
  - The lobes are connected by a band of tissue, the interthalamic adhesion, which travels through the third ventricle.
  - Both lobes help to form the caudothalamic groove inferior to the lateral ventricles bilaterally.

○ Caudate nucleus:
  - The caudate nucleus helps to form the caudothalamic groove and it is located in each cerebral hemisphere.
  - The caudate nucleus consists of a head, body, and tail.

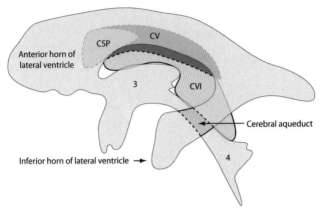

Figure 12-5. Anatomy of the cavum septum pellucidum. The cavum septum pellucidum (CSP) is a normal midline structure often noted within the premature brain. The cavum vergae (CV) and even the cavum velum interpositum (CVI) may also be noted, especially if the brain is exceedingly immature. 3, third ventricle; 4, fourth ventricle.
(Reprinted with permission from Kline-Fath B, Bahado-Singh R, Bulas D, eds. *Fundamental and Advanced Fetal Imaging.* 1st ed. Philadelphia, PA: Wolters Kluwer; 2015.)

○ Caudothalamic groove:
  – The caudothalamic groove is the bilateral groove created by the caudate nucleus and thalamus.
  – The caudothalamic groove contains the germinal matrix and is the most common location for cerebral hemorrhage to occur within the premature brain **(Fig. 12-6)**.
○ Germinal matrix:
  – The germinal matrix is a group of thin-walled blood vessels that are highly prone to rupture when a compromise to cerebral blood pressure occurs.
  – The bilateral germinal matrix is larger in preterm infants, but ultimately regresses in size to be located at the head of the caudate nucleus in the caudothalamic groove.
  – The germinal matrix is the most common location for intracranial hemorrhage to occur in the premature infant brain.

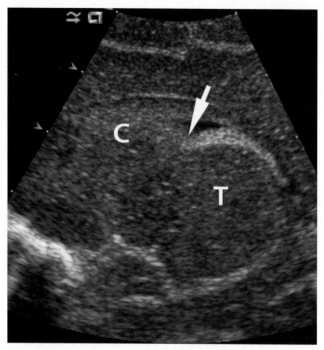

Figure 12-6. Caudothalamic groove. Magnified sonographic parasagittal scan at the level of the caudothalamic groove. Head of the caudate nucleus (C) is seen anterior to the thalamus (T). Between these two structures is the caudothalamic groove (*arrow*), which contains the anterior extent of the choroid plexus. (Reprinted with permission from Kawamura D, Nolan T, eds. *Abdomen and Superficial Structures*. 4th ed. Philadelphia, PA: Wolters Kluwer; 2017.)

- Physiology:
  - The premature infant lacks the ability to autoregulate cerebral blood pressure, and thus the brain may suffer from a lack of oxygen.
  - Lack of oxygen to the brain can result in a hypoxic–ischemic event, leading to hemorrhage and death of the affected tissue.
  - Sonography provides a noninvasive imaging modality that can assess the infant brain for signs of hemorrhage, congenital brain malformations, and other pathology.

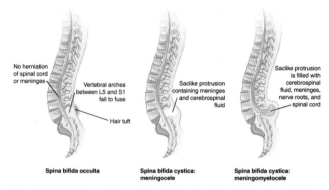

No herniation of spinal cord or meninges

Vertebral arches between L5 and S1 fail to fuse

Hair tuft

Saclike protrusion containing meninges and cerebrospinal fluid

Saclike protrusion is filled with cerebrospinal fluid, meninges, nerve roots, and spinal cord

Spina bifida occulta   **Spina bifida cystica: meningocele**   **Spina bifida cystica: meningomyelocele**

Figure 12-7. Malformation of the distal spine. (Reprinted with permission from Bowden V, Greenberg CS, eds. *Children and Their Families*. 3rd ed. Philadelphia, PA: Wolters Kluwer Health/Lippincott Williams & Wilkins; 2013.)

- Anatomy and physiology of the neonatal spine[4,5]:
  - When clinical findings are worrisome for spinal dysraphisms, the distal neonatal spine can be well demonstrated with sonography in the newborn up until around 3 mo.
  - Open spinal defects are typically visually demonstrated, while occult (hidden) lesions often require imaging (**Fig. 12-7**).
  - Overlying skin abnormalities suggestive of occult abnormalities include a sacral dimple, tuft of hair or skin tags, dorsal dermal sinus, or skin lesion such as a hemangioma located over the distal spine region.
  - Of main concern is the location of the distal spinal cord, a structure referred to as the conus medullaris (**Fig. 12-8**).
  - The conus medullaris is the tapering of the spinal cord and it should normally terminate between L1 and L2.
  - The conus medullaris gives rise to the filum terminale, which is surrounded by the cauda equine.
  - Tethering of the cord can be demonstrated with sonography when the conus medullaris is located at or below the L3 vertebral level.
  - Tethering of the cord can lead to nerve damage, and if surgical intervention is not performed, possible complications include bladder, bowel, and lower limb dysfunction.

12. Pediatrics

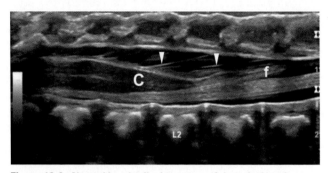

Figure 12-8. Normal longitudinal anatomy of the spinal cord.
Longitudinal scan through the distal cord shows a normal smoothly
tapering conus medullaris (C), nerve roots (*arrowheads*), and the
filum terminale (f). The second lumbar vertebral body is labeled
(L2). The conus medullaris is in a normal position at L2 to L3.
(Reprinted with permission from Siegel MJ, ed. *Pediatric Sonography*. 5th ed.
Philadelphia, PA: Wolters Kluwer; 2018.)

PATIENT PREPARATION FOR SONOGRAPHY OF THE INFANT HIP, NEONATAL BRAIN, AND NEONATAL SPINE[1-6]

- Infant hips:
  - A hip ultrasound is not typically performed on patients younger than 6 wks of age unless indicated based on abnormal findings on physical exam. Also, sonography is most useful for infants younger than 6 mo secondary to the increased ossification of the bones in older infants.
  - The optimal time to assess the infant's hips is immediately following feeding when the infant is relaxed and cooperative.
  - Rolled towels or perhaps a small-angled sponge may be needed in order to stabilize the infant when decubitus imaging is warranted.
  - Clothing should be removed from the waist down, though the diaper should remain in place.
  - Keeping the infant warm is beneficial, as well as the aid that a parent or assistant can provide during the examination.
  - A physical examination can be conducted by a *qualified examiner* prior to the sonographic examination (**Fig. 12-9**). There are two tests that are often utilized:

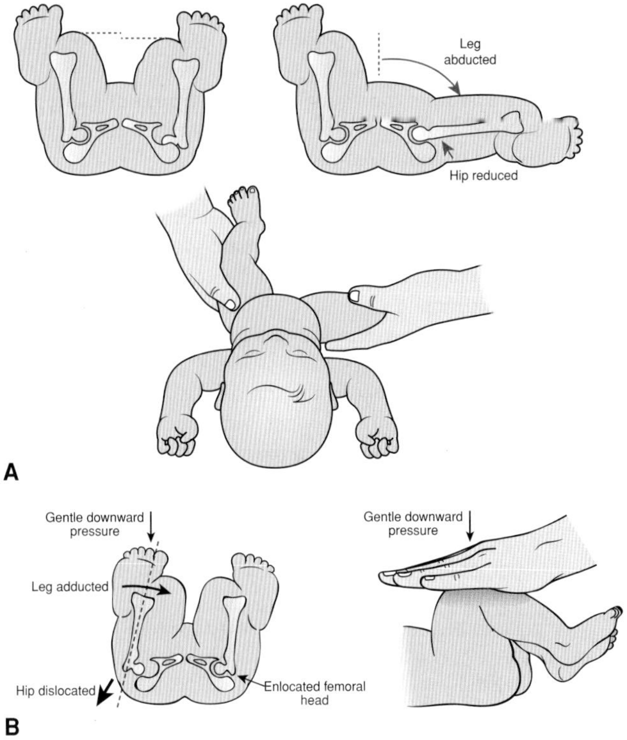

A

B

Figure 12-9. A: The Ortolani maneuver. From a flexed and adduced position, the hip is abducted; the examiner feels a clunk as the femoral head moves into the socket. The examiner's other hand stabilizes the infant's pelvis. B: The Barlow test. The examiner holds the infant's hip in flexion and slight abduction. The infant's hip is adduced while applying pressure in a posterior direction. Dislocation of the femoral head with pressure indicates an unstable hip. (Reprinted with permission from Penny S, ed. *Examination Review for Ultrasound: Abdomen and Obstetrics and Gynecology.* 2nd ed. Philadelphia, PA: Wolters Kluwer; 2017.)

- Barlow test—assesses the hip for dislocation:
  - The infant is placed in the supine position and the leg is flexed 90 degrees.
  - The examiner then grasps the symphysis pubis and sacrum with one hand, while the other hand adducts the hip by manipulating the knee.
  - Slight outward pressure is then exerted over the knee and distal thigh.
  - If the hip is dislocatable, a palpable sensation referred to as a clunk, will be felt as the femoral head exits the acetabulum.
- Ortolani test—the examiner attempts to reduce a recently dislocated hip:
  - The infant is placed in the supine position.
  - The index and middle fingers are placed along the outer femur at the level of the greater trochanter and the thumb is placed along the inner thigh.
  - The hip is then flexed 90 degrees and is then abducted while simultaneously lifting the leg anteriorly.
  - A palpable clunk is felt as the hip is reduced into the acetabulum.
  - An audible click may also be heard as well.
- A basic visual assessment can be conducted as well (Fig. 12-10):
  - Assess for signs of asymmetry in the lengths of the legs. DDH can be suspected when the knees are flexed, and one knee is notably lower than the other, thus demonstrating a leg length discrepancy.
  - Assess for signs of asymmetry in the thigh skin folds. The affected side will have both asymmetric thigh and gluteal folds.
- Neonatal brain:
  - Premature infants are often analyzed in the neonatal intensive care unit:
    - Make sure the ultrasound machine and all equipment are thoroughly cleaned.
    - Be aware that units will most likely require surgical hand asepsis before entering and providing patient care to premature infants.

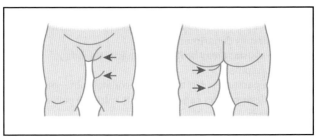

A

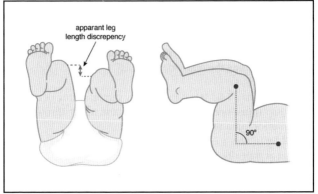

B

Figure 12-10. DDH physical findings. A: Asymmetric skin folds.
B: Leg length discrepancy. (Reprinted with permission from Sanders RC,
ed. *Clinical Sonography: A Practical Guide.* 5th ed. Philadelphia, PA: Wolters
Kluwer; 2015.)

- Work to maintain a clean environment and to not disrupt
  the infants environment too much, including maintaining
  a warm atmosphere.
- Obtain necessary information regarding the birth weight
  and current weight of the infant. Also, obtain the age of
  gestation at the time of birth and current age prior to the
  examination. This information may be provided on the
  sonographic images.

12. Pediatrics

- Evaluation of inpatient and outpatient term infants and follow-up examinations are typically performed in the sonography department:
  - An assistant may be helpful to pacify the infant.
- Neonatal spine:
  - No preparation is required for a neonatal spine sonogram.
  - A bottle or pacifier can be helpful to calm the patient during the exam.

SUGGESTED EQUIPMENT[1-5]

- Infant hips:
  - Birth to 3 mo = 7.5 MHz high-frequency linear transducer or higher
  - Older infants = 5 MHz linear transducer may be warranted
  - An assistant would be helpful for stabilizing the infant or manipulating the machine controls
- Neonatal brain:
  - Newborns = 7.5 MHz phased array vector, sector, or curved linear transducer that can fit within and image through the anterior fontanelle
  - Older infants = 5 MHz phased array vector, sector, or curved linear transducer may be warranted
  - Linear transducer may be warranted for the assessment of the superior sagittal sinus
  - The Doppler power output should be as low as reasonably achievable
- Neonatal spine:
  - Neonates = 9–12 MHz high-frequency linear array transducer
  - Older infants = 5–9 MHz high-frequency linear array transducer:
    - 3–9 MHz curvilinear transducer with a larger field of view may be helpful in larger infants
  - Transducers settings that can provide a panoramic view or a split or dual screen can be helpful
  - A towel may be warranted to elevate the abdomen in order to decrease the natural curvature of the distal spine

CLINICAL INVESTIGATION FOR SONOGRAPHY OF THE INFANT HIPS, NEONATAL BRAIN, AND NEONATAL SPINE

- Infant hips:
  - Evaluate prior imaging reports and images including previous perinatal sonogram reports for evidence of predisposing conditions such as breech position or oligohydramnios.
  - Evaluate previous radiography examinations of the hip.
  - Critical clinical history questions related to infant hips:
    - Was the baby in a breech position at the time of delivery? *A breech delivery increases the chances for the infant to suffer from DDH.*
    - Was there evidence of abnormal fetal position or oligohydramnios? *Oligohydramnios increases the chances for the infant to suffer from DDH.*
    - Any family history of DDH? *Family history increases the chances for the infant to suffer from DDH.*
    - Did the physician hear a click or pop on physical exam? *Physician examination of infants suffering from DDH could reveal an audible pop or click emanating from the abnormal hip joint.*
    - Does the infant have signs of asymmetry in the lengths of the legs? *Asymmetry in the legs can be a physical sign of DDH.*
    - Does the infant have signs of asymmetry in the thigh skin folds? *Asymmetry of the skin folds can be a physical sign of DDH.*
- Neonatal brain:
  - Evaluate prior imaging reports and images including previous perinatal sonogram reports for evidence of congenital brain abnormalities or complicated perinatal conditions.
  - Critical clinical history questions related to the neonatal brain:
    - Premature neonatal brain:
      - What was the gestational age at the time of birth? *Preterm infants who are born less than 32 wks of gestational age are at high-risk for suffering from intracranial hemorrhage.*

- ○ What was the birth weight? *Preterm infants who are born weighing <1,500 g are at high risk for suffering from intracranial hemorrhage.*
- ○ What is the current age of the infant? *Oftentimes, intracranial hemorrhage may not be visualized with sonography until 3–4 d after birth.*
- Mature infant brain:
  - ○ Was the infant born prematurely? *A history of prematurity increases the risk for intracranial hemorrhage.*
  - ○ Is the infant feeding normally? *Hydrocephalus and congenital brain anomalies can cause associated feeding issues in infants.*
  - ○ Is the head enlarged? *Pediatricians measure the head circumference in the neonatal period to assess for signs of hydrocephalus.*
- Neonatal spine:
  - Evaluate prior imaging reports and images including previous postnatal radiography exams.
  - Critical clinical history questions related to the neonatal spine:
    - Does the infant have any skin features or external defects suggestive of a spinal dysraphism? *Overlying skin abnormalities suggestive of occult abnormalities include a sacral dimple, tuft of hair or skin tags, dorsal dermal sinus, or skin lesion such as a hemangioma located over the distal spine region.*
    - Are there any perinatal sonographic findings suggestive of spina bifida? *Open neural tube defects may be discovered in utero and thus obstetric sonogram reports should be obtained if possible.*

NORMAL SONOGRAPHIC DESCRIPTION OF INFANT HIPS, NEONATAL BRAIN, AND NEONATAL SPINE[1-4]

- Infant hips:
  - The femoral head appears as a hypoechoic well-circumscribed circle containing hyperechoic dots (Fig. 12-11).
  - The femoral neck is hyperechoic and extends medially, superiorly, and anteriorly as it tapers toward the head of the femur.

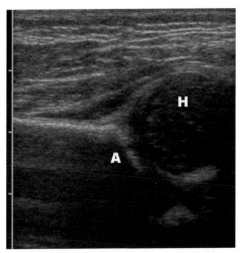

Figure 12-11. Normal neonatal hip in coronal. The femoral head (H) is clearly distinguishable as a hypoechoic round structure containing multiple hyperechoic foci. It is noted within the curved hyperechoic cup-shaped acetabulum (A). (Reprinted with permission from Chew FS, ed. *Skeletal Radiology.* 3rd ed. Philadelphia, PA: Wolters Kluwer Health/Lippincott Williams & Wilkins; 2010.)

- The acetabulum is a cup-shaped hyperechoic fossa that should contain the femoral head.
- The labrum is best seen in coronal as a triangular hypoechoic structure adjacent to the ileum and superolateral to the femoral head.
- The ileum is hyperechoic and produces an acoustic shadow.
- Neonatal brain:
  - The mid-low level echoes that comprise the brain parenchyma in the premature infant may appear exceedingly smooth, lacking sulci and gyri. As the infant brain matures more sulci and gyri can be noted (Fig. 12-12).
  - Sulci and gyri appear as hyperechoic curvilinear structures that course throughout the mature brain parenchyma.
  - The normal lateral ventricles appear as slit-like structures in the mature infant brain, while in the premature brain the ventricles are much more prominent and slightly distended with anechoic CSF.

12. Pediatrics

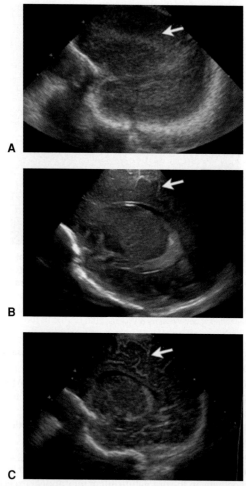

Figure 12-12. Normal neonatal brain and mature brain sonographic features. Parasagittal US images of normal 26-wk (A), normal 35-wk (B), and normal term (C) infants. Head sonography is the most frequent means of neonatal brain imaging. Note how sulcation (*arrows*) evolves from a smooth cortical mantle at 26 wk (A), into a highly organized adult pattern by term (C) (*arrows*). (Reprinted with permission from Brant WE, Helms C, eds. *Fundamentals of Diagnostic Radiology.* 4th ed. Philadelphia, PA: Wolters Kluwer Health/Lippincott Williams & Wilkins; 2012.)

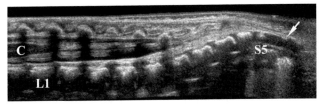

Figure 12-13. Normal infant spine, extended field of view.
Longitudinal extended field-of-view image in a newborn infant
shows the entire lower spinal cord and its relationship to the
spine. S5 is the first ossified vertebral segment, the coccyx (*arrow*) is
unossified, and the conus (C) ends normally at L1–L2. (Reprinted with
permission from Siegel MJ, ed. *Pediatric Sonography.* 4th ed. Philadelphia,
PA: Wolters Kluwer Health/Lippincott Williams & Wilkins; 2010.)

- The CSP can be noted in the midline of the brain. In
  the premature infant, a posterior extension of the CSP
  referred to as the cavum vergae, can be identified as well.
  Occasionally, the cavum interpositum can be seen as an
  anechoic structure inferior to the cavum vergae.
- The bilateral caudothalamic grooves can be noted as
  hyperechoic curvilinear structures located between the
  caudate nuclei and lobes of the thalamus.
- Bilateral sylvian fissure can also be noted laterally as
  echogenic curvilinear structures.
- Neonatal spine:
  - In longitudinal, the spinal cord appears as a hypoechoic
    tubular structure with anterior and posterior borders that
    should ultimately taper at the conus medullaris, typically
    at the level of the first or second lumbar vertebral body
    (Fig. 12-13).
  - The echogenic central complex can be noted within the
    spinal cord.
  - Anechoic CSF is located within the anterior subarachnoid
    space and should be seen adjacent to the spinal cord.
  - The echogenic vertebral bodies can be noted anterior to
    the spinal cord, while the echogenic posterior elements
    of the spine are noted posteriorly.
  - The spinal cord is bordered posteriorly by the hypoechoic
    cartilaginous spinous processes, hyperechoic dura mater,
    and CSF-filled posterior subarachnoid space.

12. Pediatrics

- The conus medullaris gives rise to the fibrous filum terminale, which should extend into the distal sacral canal.
- Upon real-time investigation, the spinal cord should be noted freely moving within the spinal canal.
- In transverse, the spinal cord appears as a hypoechoic oval or round structure with an echogenic central complex.
- Nerve fibers that extend from the spinal cord can be noted as hyperechoic linear structures coursing away from the cord and filum terminale.

SUGGESTED PROTOCOL FOR SONOGRAPHY OF INFANT HIPS, NEONATAL BRAIN, AND NEONATAL SPINE[1–6]

- Infant hips:
  - Both hips should be examined with sonography.
  - If possible, some type of pacification for the infant should be provided, including feeding the infant during the exam to minimize irritability.
  - Each hip can be examined in the supine or related decubitus positions.
  - Each hip is examined in coronal at rest and transverse with and without stress.
  - Careful labeling should be maintained to include "stress" and/or "neutral."
    - Coronal view **(Fig. 12-14) (Video 12-1)**
  - The anatomic coronal image is obtained by manipulating the superior edge of the transducer 10–15 degrees into an oblique coronal image in order for the ilium to appear straight. This will provide a longitudinal image of the hip.
  - The iliac line will be noted superiorly and the femoral neck will be noted inferiorly in the image.
  - In the coronal/neutral scan plane, the leg can be extended or remain in the neutral position.
  - Both alpha and beta angle can be obtained in the coronal plane **(Fig. 12-15)**.
    - Graf technique—measurement of the relationship between the acetabulum and the femoral head.
      - Three lines and two angles are drawn around the acetabulum.

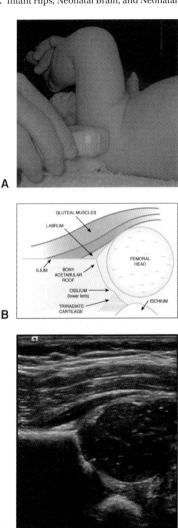

Figure 12-14. **Coronal infant hip. A: Probe placement on an infant hip for the coronal flexion view. Please note the infant's knee is bent at approximately 90 degrees. B: Anatomic drawing of the infant hip in coronal. C: Normal coronal sonogram of the infant hip in the coronal plane.** (Reprinted with permission from Sanders RC, ed. *Clinical Sonography: A Practical Guide*. 5th ed. Philadelphia, PA: Wolters Kluwer; 2015.)

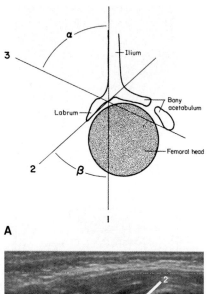

A

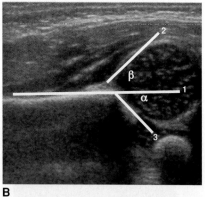

B

Figure 12-15. **The Graf technique. Drawing of the coronal view of the hip (A) and coronal sonogram (B) delineate the femoral head, bony acetabulum, and labrum. A horizontal baseline is drawn along the ilium (1), along with lines along the labrum (2) and bony acetabulum (3). The alpha angle measures the acetabulum and is equal to greater than 60 degrees in infants with seated hips and less than 50 degrees in patients with dysplasia.** (Panel A adapted by permission from the Springer: Graf R. Classification of hip joint dysplasia by means of sonography. *Arch Orthop Trauma Surg.* 1984;102(4);248–255. Copyright © 1984 Springer Nature; Panel B reprinted with permission from Siegel MJ, ed. *Pediatric Sonography.* 4th ed. Philadelphia, PA: Wolters Kluwer Health/Lippincott Williams & Wilkins; 2010.)

- – Alpha angle:
  - Obtained by drawing one line along the straight edge of the iliac bone and a second line along the bony acetabular roof.
- – Beta angle:
  - Obtained by drawing one line through the straight edge of the iliac bone and a line through the echogenic fibrocartilaginous labrum.
- ○ Coverage of the femoral head by the acetabulum should also be assessed.
- ○ Validation by angle and femoral head coverage measurement is optional. Performance of stress in this plane is also optional.
- Transverse:
  - ○ The correct transverse plane is the anatomic transverse or axial plane with respect to the body (**Fig. 12-16**).
  - ○ Flexion position is adequate, though some may prefer to include a neutral position also.
  - ○ Transverse flexion is made from a transverse plane with the femur flexed 90 degrees.
  - ○ The femoral shaft and ischium should form a U or V configuration with the femoral head.
  - ○ Stress maneuvers can be performed in real time to assess the seating position of the femoral head into the acetabulum (**Video 12-2**). 🎬
  - ○ Stress maneuvers are not performed when the hips are being examined in a Pavlik harness or split device unless otherwise specified.
- Neonatal brain:
  - The brain should be examined with the infant in the supine position, though it may be in the prone position if needed.
  - Transducer orientation is critical, so ensure that in coronal the index or notch is located on the right side of the head, while in sagittal the notch should be positioned anteriorly.
    - Coronal images should include (**Figs. 12-17 and 12-18**) (**Video 12-3**): 🎬
      - ○ Frontal lobes anterior to the frontal horns of the lateral ventricles with orbits visualized deep to the skull base.
      - ○ Frontal horns or bodies of the lateral ventricles and interhemispheric fissure.

12. Pediatrics

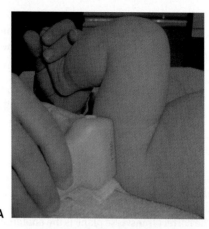

A

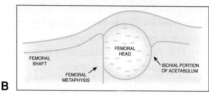

B

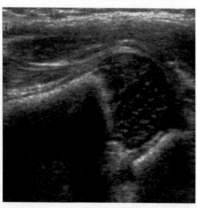

C

Figure 12-16. **Transverse infant hip. A: Transducer placement for flexion transverse imaging of the infant hip. B: Drawing of the infant hip anatomy in the transverse flexion view. C: Sonogram of the normal infant hip in transverse.** (Reprinted with permission from Sanders RC, ed. *Clinical Sonography: A Practical Guide.* 5th ed. Philadelphia, PA: Wolters Kluwer; 2015.)

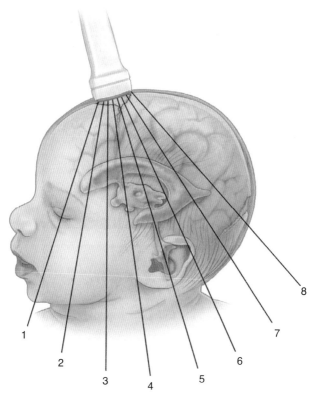

Figure 12-17. Transducer placement and manipulation for coronal imaging of the neonatal brain. Note that the transducer notch or index is placed on the patient's right side. (Reprinted with permission from Kawamura D, Nolan T, eds. *Abdomen and Superficial Structures.* 4th ed. Philadelphia, PA: Wolters Kluwer; 2017.)

- ○ Lateral ventricles at the level of the lateral and third ventricles.
- ○ Include interhemispheric fissure, cingulate sulcus (if developed), corpus callosum, septum pellucidum or cavum septi pellucidi, caudate nuclei, putamina, globi pallidi, and sylvian fissures. The foramina of Monro should also be depicted, outlining the course of the choroid plexus from the lateral into the third ventricle.

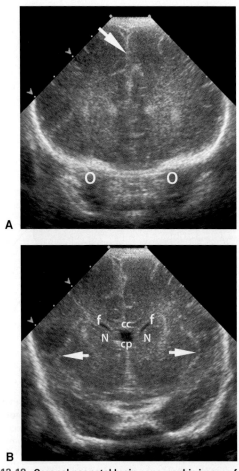

Figure 12-18. Coronal neonatal brain sonographic images from anterior to posterior. A: Image of the frontal lobes includes the interhemispheric fissure (*white arrow*). The orbital ridges (O) are also noted. B: The frontal horns (f) appear as triangular-shaped, fluid-filled spaces separated by the cavum septum pellucidum (cp). The head of the caudate nuclei (N) lie adjacent to the lateral walls of the ventricles. The hypoechoic corpus callosum (cc) forms the roof of the cavum. The echogenic Y-shaped sylvian fissures (*arrows*) are seen laterally.

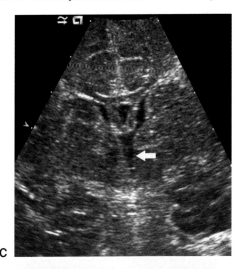

C

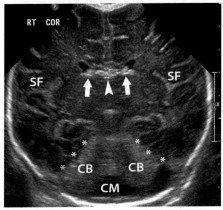

D

Figure 12-18 *(continued)*. C: Magnified coronal image at the level of the normal third ventricle. Slight off-axis scan shows the normal size third ventricle (*arrow*) at the level of the foramen of Monro. D: The echogenic choroid plexus is seen in the floor of the lateral ventricles (*arrows*) and the roof of the third ventricle (*arrowhead*). The Y-shaped sylvian fissures (SF) are seen laterally. Also visible are the echogenic tentorium (*asterisk*), the cerebellar hemispheres (CB), and the cisterna magna (CM). *(continued)*

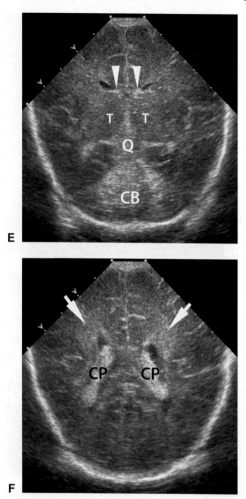

Figure 12-18 *(continued).* E: Coronal image taken at the level of the quadrigeminal cistern. The star-shaped echogenic quadrigeminal cistern (Q) is seen inferior to the thalami (T). The cerebellum (CB) and the echogenic choroid plexus (*arrowhead*) in the floor of the lateral ventricles are also visualized on this image. F: Coronal scan at the level of the trigones of the lateral ventricles. The largest part of the choroid plexus (CP), the glomus, can be seen occupying most of the lateral ventricles. The periventricular matter is located lateral to the ventricles (*arrows*).

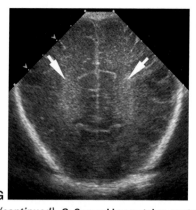

G

Figure 12-18 *(continued)*. **G: Coronal image taken posterior to the occipital horns of lateral ventricles shows the normal echogenic periventricular white matter (*arrows*) and the occipital cortex.**
(Reprinted with permission from Kawamura D, Nolan T, eds. *Abdomen and Superficial Structures*. 4th ed. Philadelphia, PA: Wolters Kluwer; 2017.)

○ Lateral ventricles slightly posterior to the foramina of Monro where the lateral and third ventricles communicate. Include the pons and medulla, thalami, and choroid plexus in the roof of the third ventricle and in the caudothalamic grooves.
○ Level of the quadrigeminal cistern and cerebellum. Include the cerebellar vermis, cisterna magna posteriorly and inferiorly, bodies of the lateral ventricles bordered by caudate nuclei and thalami, and temporal horns.
○ Echogenic glomi of choroid plexuses at the posterior aspect of the lateral ventricles at the level of trigones. Include the splenium of the corpus callosum at divergence of the lateral ventricle, periventricular white matter lateral to posterior horns of the lateral ventricles.
○ Area posterior to the occipital horns. Include parietal and occipital lobes and the posterior interhemispheric fissure.
○ Additional coronal image:
  – Extra-axial fluid spaces as needed. Use linear high-frequency (≥9 MHz) transducers to obtain a coronal

12. Pediatrics

magnification view of the extra-axial fluid space, including only peripheral brain structures (superior sagittal sinus at the level of the frontal horns; measure the sinocortical distance, craniocortical distance, and width of the interhemispheric fissure).

- Sagittal images should include (**Figs. 12-19 and 12-20**) (**Video 12-4**):
  - Midline sagittal view to include the corpus callosum, cavum septum pellucidi, and cavum vergae if present, third and fourth ventricles, cerebral aqueduct, brain stem, cerebellar vermis, cisterna magna, and sulci.
  - Bilateral parasagittal images to include all parts of the lateral ventricles, the choroid plexus, caudothalamic grooves, insula, periventricular white matter, and sylvian fissures.
- Additional views and images:
  - Mastoid views and posterior views may be utilized to demonstrate the cerebellum and posterior elements of the brain.
  - Pulsed Doppler assessment of the resistive index of the midline anterior cerebral artery may be obtained.
  - A color Doppler linear image of the anterior surface of the brain may be obtained to evaluate for subdural hemorrhage. Normal subarachnoid fluid has crossing vessels (cortical vein sign), whereas abnormal subdural fluid does not.
- Neonatal spine:
  - The examination is usually performed with the infant lying in the prone position, although the study can also be done with the patient in the decubitus position.
  - A small bolster may be placed under the lower abdomen or pelvis to mildly flex the back, which may improve imaging.
  - The knees may be flexed to improve visualization of the spinal canal.
  - The infant should be kept warm and pacified.
  - Images are typically obtained in the longitudinal and transverse scan planes.
  - Extended field-of view images or landscape views are highly beneficial.
  - Cine clips can be used to demonstrate cord motion and provide an overall view of the spine (**Video 12-5**).

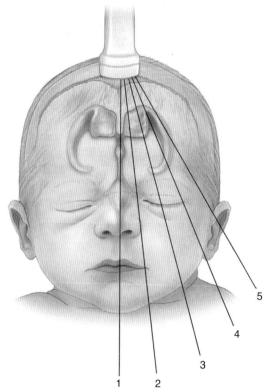

Figure 12-19. Transducer placement for imaging of the neonatal brain in the sagittal and parasagittal plane. Note that the transducer notch or index is placed toward the patient's face. (Reprinted with permission from Kawamura D, Nolan T, eds. *Abdomen and Superficial Structures.* 4th ed. Philadelphia, PA: Wolters Kluwer; 2017.)

- Longitudinal spine
  - Studies may be limited to the lumbosacral region in specific cases, as in those patients being evaluated for a sacrococcygeal dimple and tethered cord.
  - Normal cord morphology and the level of termination of the conus should be assessed and documented, which requires accurate identification of vertebral body level.

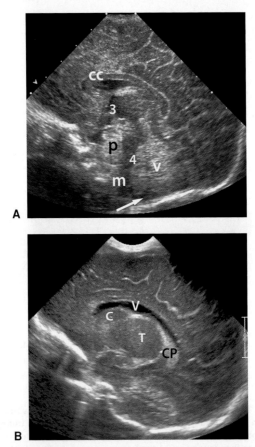

Figure 12-20. Sagittal and parasagittal neonatal brain sonographic images. A: Sagittal midline. Normal midline sagittal image on a term infant. The hypoechoic corpus callosum (cc) is seen anterior to the cavum septum pellucidum. The third (3) and fourth (4) ventricles are visible in this plane. Posterior to the fourth ventricle is the echogenic vermis of the cerebellum (v) and the cisterna magna (*arrow*). Anterior to the fourth ventricle is the pons (p) and medulla (m). B: Parasagittal scan through the area of the lateral ventricle. The highly echogenic choroid plexus (CP) is seen within the body of the lateral ventricle (V) and tapers to a point at the caudothalamic groove. The caudate nucleus (C) anterior to the thalamus (T) is again noted. This is the location of the germinal matrix in premature infants.

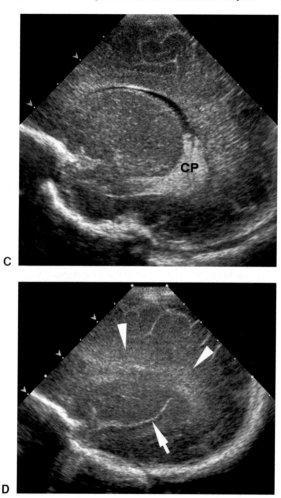

C

D

Figure 12-20 *(continued)*. C: Parasagittal scan through the body of the lateral ventricle. The echogenic choroid plexus (CP) is seen within the trigone of the ventricle. D: Parasagittal scan lateral to the ventricle. The sylvian fissure (*arrow*) is seen in this scan, and on real-time scanning, the branches of the middle cerebral arteries can be seen pulsating within this fissure. Normal periventricular white matter (*arrowheads*) lateral to the ventricle. (Reprinted with permission from Kawamura D, Nolan T, eds. *Abdomen and Superficial Structures*. 4th ed. Philadelphia, PA: Wolters Kluwer; 2017.)

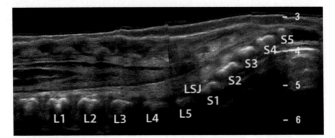

Figure 12-21. Lumbosacral junction. This longitudinal image of the distal infant spine depicts the vertebral column and the lumbosacral junction, which is a crucial landmark used to help count the vertebral bodies and to determine the location of the conus. (Reprinted with permission from Kawamura D, Lunsford B, eds. *Abdomen and Superficial Structures.* 3rd ed. Philadelphia, PA: Wolters Kluwer Health/Lippincott Williams & Wilkins; 2012.)

- Method 1:
  - Identification of the normal lumbosacral curvature to locate the lumbosacral junction and thus the location of L5 is a means to determine the location of the conus (**Fig. 12-21**).
  - The vertebral level of the conus medullaris is then determined by counting cephalad from L5.
  - Extended field-of-view (panoramic) imaging can often aid in identification of a longer segment of the spine and facilitate identification of the vertebral level.
  - The first coccygeal segment may or may not be ossified at birth, though it can be differentiated by its rounder shape compared to the rectangular shape of the sacral bodies.
- Method 2:
  - The last rib-bearing vertebra can be presumed to be T12, and the lumbar level of the conus can then be determined by counting from superior to inferior of the successive vertebral bodies.
  - The conus is normally located at or above the L2 to L3 disk space. However, a normal conus located at the mid-L3 level may be identified, especially in preterm infants; this position is considered the lower limits of normal.

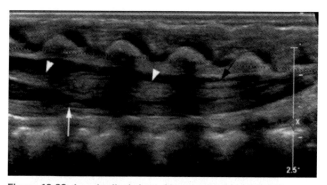

Figure 12-22. Longitudinal view of lower spinal canal showing echogenic roots of cauda equina (*arrowheads*). Distal cord tapers into conus (*white arrow*). Filum terminale (*black arrow*) extends from conus to distal thecal sac. (Reprinted with permission from Iyer R, Chapman T, eds. *Pediatric Imaging: The Essentials.* 1st ed. Philadelphia, PA: Wolters Kluwer; 2015.)

- ○ Cord motion should be noted with respiration and the cord should rest anteriorly in the spinal canal when the patient is in the prone position. A motionless spinal cord may be suggestive of a tethered cord.
- ○ The filum of the cord and its thickness should be noted (**Fig. 12-22**).
- ○ Abnormal fluid collections in and around the cord should be noted.
- ○ Tracts extending from the skin surface should be assessed for connection into the spinal canal.
- ○ A stand-off pad or a thick layer of coupling gel may be used, if needed, to evaluate the superficial soft tissues and skin line for the presence of a tract.
- ● Transverse spine (**Fig. 12-23**):
  - ○ Transverse images are essential to identify and document diastematomyelia (split spinal cord).
  - ○ Open posterior elements in skin-covered dysraphic defects can be documented on transverse views.
  - ○ The filum of the cord and its thickness should be noted.

12. Pediatrics

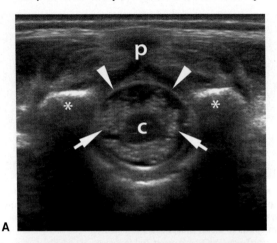

A

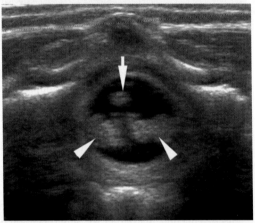

B

Figure 12-23. Normal transverse spinal cord. A: The hypoechoic spinal cord (c) is surrounded by the echogenic nerve roots of the cauda equina (*arrows*). Cerebrospinal fluid surrounds the cord that is contained by the echogenic dura (*arrowheads*) encompassing the canal. Echogenic vertebral arches (*) are noted posterior and laterally joining with the hypoechoic spinous process (p) posteriorly. B: A slightly more prominent echogenic round filum terminale (*arrow*) floats among echogenic nerve roots (*arrowheads*).

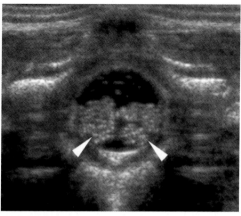

C

Figure 12-23 *(continued).* **C: Nerve roots can appear as small echogenic dots (*arrowheads*) or clump together, sometimes obscuring the filum terminale.** (Reprinted with permission from Kawamura D, Nolan T, eds. *Abdomen and Superficial Structures.* 4th ed. Philadelphia, PA: Wolters Kluwer; 2017.)

SCANNING TIPS[4]

- Infant hips:
  - False-positive results for DDH can result from improper transducer orientation of the acetabulum with the femoral head and triradiate cartilage. To correct improper orientation in the coronal view, ensure that the beam is centered over the acetabulum and that the ilium is parallel to the transducer face.
  - Scanning at 6 wks may not always be helpful because the immature acetabulum may be underdeveloped. Thus, inconclusive or indeterminate exams should be followed up.
  - Acoustic shadowing produced by the femoral head or acetabulum can prohibit the complete visualization of the hip joint. Thus, a radiographic examination may be warranted.
- Neonatal brain:
  - Asymmetry between the lateral ventricles may be noted. In most cases, the larger ventricle is the side that the infant is lying on and this is secondary to that ventricle becoming distended with more CSF due to gravity.

12. Pediatrics

- The "three dot sign" is the sonographic sign of choroid plexus located in the roof of the third ventricle and the floor of both lateral ventricles. This sign can simulate bilateral germinal matrix hemorrhages.
- The normal periventricular halo can appear similar to periventricular leukomalacia. However, the tissue containing the normal halo should not appear brighter than the choroid plexus.
- Neonatal spine:
  - Two other methods exist for determining the location of the conus:
    - The thecal sac usually ends at S2. This level can then be used to count cephalad to determine the location of the conus.
    - When the level of the conus cannot be definitively assessed as normal or abnormal, correlation with previous plain radiographs, if available, is helpful. A radiopaque marker can be placed on the skin at the level of the conus determined sonographically, followed by an anterior–posterior spine radiograph.

NORMAL MEASUREMENTS OF INFANT HIPS, NEONATAL BRAIN, AND NEONATAL SPINE[4,5]

- Infant hips:
  - Graf technique:
    - Alpha angle is normally ≥60 degrees:
      - The smaller the alpha angle, the more likely DDH is present.
    - Beta angle is normally ≤50 degrees:
      - The greater the beta angle, the more likely DDH is present.
  - Coverage of the femoral head by the acetabulum of greater than 55% or less is normal, while less than 50% is said to be shallow, and less than 45% is said to be very shallow.
- Neonatal brain:
  - Lateral ventricles: Term infants should have slit-like lateral ventricles that measure <3 mm in diameter.
- Neonatal spine:
  - Normal conus medullaris is nearly always located above the L2–L3 disc space.
  - Filum terminale thickness ≤2 mm.
  - Lumbar portion of the cord = 5.8 ± 0.66 mm.

ESSENTIAL PATHOLOGY OF INFANT HIPS, NEONATAL BRAIN, AND NEONATAL SPINE[5–7]

- Infant hips:
  - Developmental dysplasia of the infant hip:
    - Clinical findings:
      - History of breech birth
      - Family history of DDH
      - Asymmetric skin folds on the legs
      - Leg length discrepancy
      - Limited limb abduction
      - Positive Barlow or Ortolani test
    - Sonographic findings:
      - Complete dislocation: femoral head located completely outside of the acetabulum (Fig. 12-24)
      - Subluxation: partial coverage of the femoral head by the acetabulum (Fig. 12-25)
      - Evidence of a shallow acetabulum demonstrating <50% coverage of the femoral head
      - Small alpha angle
      - Large beta angle
  - Infant hip joint effusion (transient synovitis):
    - Clinical findings:
      - Leg and knee pain
      - Reluctance to walk
      - Irritability
      - Low-grade fever
      - Mild leukocytosis
    - Sonographic findings:
      - An anechoic or hypoechoic fluid collection that elevates the anterior capsule of the joint
      - Width of the abnormal hip joint capsule typically exceeds 5 mm
- Neonatal brain:
  - Intracranial/intraventricular hemorrhage grades:
    - Grade I = Germinal matrix hemorrhage (subependymal hemorrhage) (Fig. 12-26)
    - Grade II = Germinal matrix hemorrhage + Intraventricular hemorrhage (Fig. 12-27)

12. Pediatrics

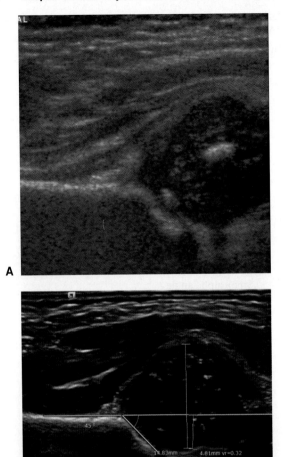

Figure 12-24. Coronal image of partial dislocation and severe acetabular dysplasia of the infant hip (A, B). (Reprinted with permission from Sanders RC, ed. *Clinical Sonography: A Practical Guide.* 5th ed. Philadelphia, PA: Wolters Kluwer; 2015.)

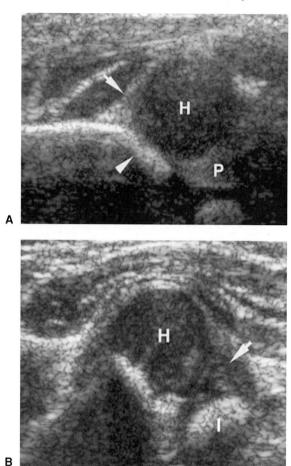

Figure 12-25. Subluxation. A: Coronal flexion views of the left hip. The femoral head (H) is positioned laterally but maintains contact with the bony acetabulum (*arrowhead*) and the labrum (*arrow*). Note the echogenic pulvinar (P) deep to the femoral head. B: Transverse flexion view. The femoral head (H) is subluxed posteriorly in relationship to the ischium (I) and acetabular roof cartilage (*arrow*). (Reprinted with permission from Siegel MJ, Coley B, eds. *Core Curriculum: Pediatric Imaging*. 1st ed. Philadelphia, PA: Lippincott Williams & Wilkins; 2005.)

12. Pediatrics

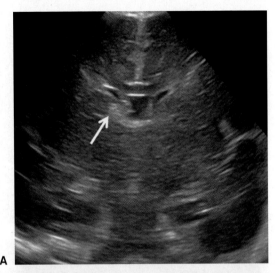

A

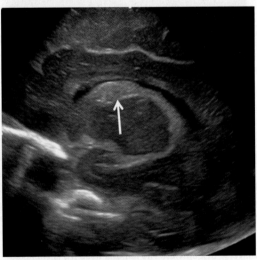

B

Figure 12-26. Germinal matrix hemorrhage (grade I). A: Coronal sonogram shows a focus of increased echogenicity (*arrow*) in the right subependymal area. B: Right parasagittal image shows increased echogenicity in the caudothalamic groove (*arrow*).
(Reprinted with permission from Siegel MJ, ed. *Pediatric Sonography*. 5th ed. Philadelphia, PA: Wolters Kluwer; 2018.)

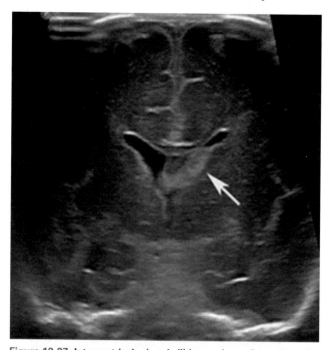

Figure 12-27. Intraventricular (grade II) hemorrhage. Coronal cranial image shows an intraventricular ovoid hemorrhage (*arrow*) within the left lateral ventricle. Note absence of ventricular dilatation.
(Reprinted with permission from Iyer R, Chapman T, eds. *Pediatric Imaging: The Essentials.* 1st ed. Philadelphia, PA: Wolters Kluwer; 2015.)

- Grade III = Intraventricular hemorrhage + Ventriculomegally **(Fig. 12-28)**
- Grade IV = Intraparenchymal hemorrhage **(Fig. 12-29)**
- Periventricular leukomalacia:
  - Stage I = Increased echogenicity of the periventricular white matter **(Fig. 12-30)**
  - Stage II = Cystic spaces form adjacent to both lateral ventricles (Fig. 12-30)

12. Pediatrics

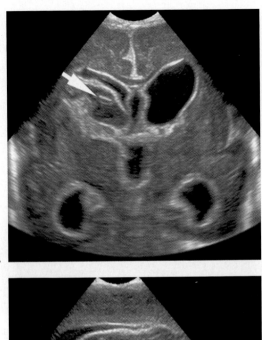

A

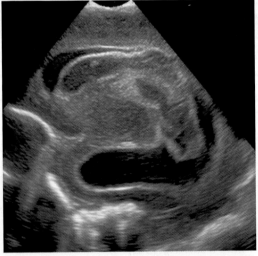

B

Figure 12-28. **Neonatal brain with intraventricular hemorrhage with ventriculomegaly (grade III). A: Coronal scan shows clot in both lateral ventricles with hydrocephalus (*arrow*). B: Parasagittal scan shows some retraction of the intraventricular clot.** (Reprinted with permission from Kawamura D, Nolan T, eds. *Abdomen and Superficial Structures.* 4th ed. Philadelphia, PA: Wolters Kluwer; 2017.)

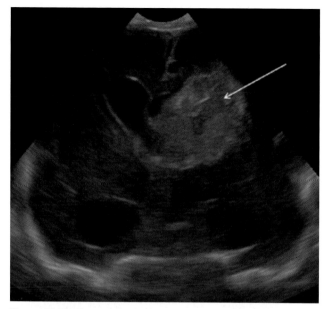

Figure 12-29. Neonatal brain with intraparenchymal hemorrhage (grade IV). An echogenic hemorrhage (*arrow*) is noted within the left lateral aspect of this neonatal brain. (Reprinted with permission from White AJ, ed. *The Washington Manual of Pediatrics*. 2nd ed. Philadelphia, PA: Wolters Kluwer; 2016.)

- Neonatal spine:
  - Tethering of the spinal cord:
    - Clinical findings:
      - Overlying skin abnormalities suggestive of occult abnormalities include a sacral dimple, tuft of hair or skin tags, dorsal dermal sinus, or skin lesion such as a hemangioma located over the distal spine region.
      - Obvious spinal external defect such as a meningomyelocele.
    - Sonographic findings:
      - Absence of the normal motion of the spinal cord.
      - Conus medullaris located at or below the L3 vertebral level **(Fig. 12-31)**.

12. Pediatrics

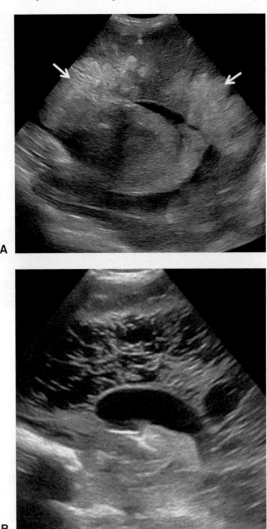

Figure 12-30. Stages of periventricular leukomalacia. A: A right parasagittal image demonstrates the echogenic pattern of periventricular leukomalacia (*arrows*) in its early stage. B: Follow-up examination reveals the later stage of periventricular leukomalacia. (Reprinted with permission from Siegel MJ, ed. *Pediatric Sonography.* 5th ed. Philadelphia, PA: Wolters Kluwer; 2018.)

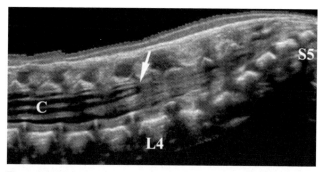

Figure 12-31. Tethering of the spinal cord. Longitudinal extended field-of-view image shows an elongated spinal cord (C) that is dorsally displaced within the thecal sac. The tip of the conus (*arrow*) is elongated and low lying at L4, indicating a tethered cord. There was no appreciable thickening of the filum and no other abnormality to account for the cord tethering. (Reprinted with permission from Siegel MJ, ed. *Pediatric Sonography.* 4th ed. Philadelphia, PA: Wolters Kluwer Health/Lippincott Williams & Wilkins; 2010.)

WHERE ELSE TO LOOK

- Infant Hips:
  - Obtaining a thorough clinical obstetric history is vital. If prenatal reports are available, evaluate for DDH-predisposing conditions.
  - Always sonographically evaluate both hips for comparison and assess the external physical signs mentioned earlier in this chapter before beginning the exam.
- Neonatal brain:
  - Note the cerebellar hemispheres for signs of asymmetry. This could be a sign of cerebellar hemorrhage.
  - Evaluate the internal components of the lateral ventricles for signs of choroid plexus bleeds and for intraventricular hemorrhage.
- Neonatal spine:
  - Urinary tract anomalies may accompany spinal dysraphisms. An assessment of the kidneys and bladder may be warranted in some cases, especially if clinical suspicions abound.

12. Pediatrics

IMAGE CORRELATION

- Infant hips radiograph of DDH **(Fig. 12-32)**
- Neonatal spine MRI with tethering of the cord **(Fig. 12-33)**

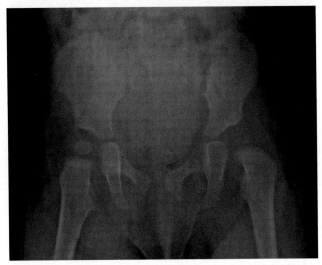

Figure 12-32. Frontal radiograph of the pelvis in a 7-mo-old girl with left DDH. (Reprinted with permission from Lee E, ed. *Pediatric Radiology: Practical Imaging Evaluation of Infants and Children.* 1st ed. Philadelphia, PA: Wolters Kluwer; 2017.)

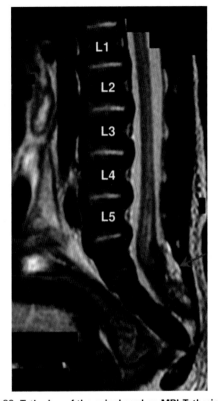

Figure 12-33. Tethering of the spinal cord on MRI. Tethering of the cord to the L5–S1 level. The spinal cord should not extend below the inferior endplate of L2. Significant spinal dysraphism with an associated 1.3-cm intraspinal lipoma (*red arrow*) is causing tethering of the cord. (Reprinted with permission from Salimpour RR, Salimpour P, Salimpour P, eds. *Photographic Atlas of Pediatric Disorders and Diagnosis.* 1st ed. Philadelphia, PA: Wolters Kluwer Health/Lippincott Williams & Wilkins; 2013.)

REFERENCES

1. AIUM-ACR-SPR-SRU Practice parameter for the performance of an ultrasound examination for detection and assessment of developmental dysplasia of the hip. https://www.aium.org/resources/guidelines/hip.pdf. Accessed December 16, 2018.

2. AIUM Practice parameter for the performance of neurosonography in neonates and infants. https://www.aium.org/resources/guidelines/neurosonography.pdf. Accessed December 16, 2018.

3. AIUM Practice parameter for the performance of an ultrasound examination of the neonatal and infant spine. https://www.aium.org/resources/guidelines/neonatalSpine.pdf. Accessed December 16, 2018.

4. Sanders R, Hall-Terracciano B, eds. *Clinical Sonography: A Practical Guide.* 5th ed. Philadelphia, PA: Wolters Kluwer; 2016:Hips 670–690;Head 626–656;Spine 657–669.

5. Siegel MJ, ed. *Pediatric Sonography.* 4th ed. Philadelphia, PA: Wolters Kluwer; 2011:Hips 607–616;Head 43–117;Spine 647–674.

6. Kawamura DM, Nolan TD, eds. *Diagnostic Medical Sonography: Abdomen and Superficial Structures.* 4th ed. Philadelphia, PA: Wolters Kluwer; 2018:687–737.

7. Penny SM, ed. *Examination Review for Ultrasound: Abdomen & Obstetrics and Gynecology.* 2nd ed. Philadelphia, PA: Wolters Kluwer; 2018:232–236.

NOTE: Page numbers followed by f indicate figures; t indicate tables.